THE Skinny on Fat

THE
Skinny
on Fat

SHAWNA VOGEL

W. H. Freeman and Company
New York

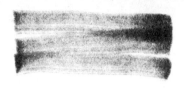

Text Design: Nancy Singer

Library of Congress Cataloging-in-Publication Data

Vogel, Shawna.
    The skinny on fat / Shawna Vogel.
        p. cm.
    Includes bibliographical references and index.
    ISBN 0-7167-3091-X
    1. Obesity   2. Weight loss.   I. Title.
RC628.V64   1999   98-43480
616.3 ' 98—dc21   CIP

Printed in the United States of America

First printing, 1999

W. H. Freeman and Company
41 Madison Avenue, New York, NY 10010
Houndmills, Basingstoke   RG21 6XS, England

FOR CONRAD

Contents

Introduction

In 1993 the American Association for the Advancement of Science sponsored a two-day seminar on advances in the field of obesity research. I sat in the audience with about a hundred other curious participants, some heavy, some not, as a half dozen scientists described their efforts to solve some of the riddles of how our bodies control weight. "Does exercise help people lose weight or just cause them to eat more?" asked one energetic researcher in silver wire-frames. "Do obese people overeat, compared to people of average weight?" the next speaker intoned during his opening remarks.

At one point during the first morning's talks, two researchers began to debate whether encouraging people to eat slowly helps them to eat less overall, and my mind drifted away from their arguments to the sound of my mother's voice. "Chew slowly," she used to say. "Drink lots of water." "Eat six small meals a day instead of three large ones." As a lifelong dieter, my mother went through every regime recommended by the experts and many that had not been: the all-watermelon diet, high-protein shakes, the benefits of vinegar. All were part of her education in dieting, and over the years these experiences had become a suit of armor in her endless struggle to take off and keep off about a dozen unwanted pounds.

As I sat in a hotel conference room listening to researchers talk about different approaches to treatment, I began to get the feeling that scientific research on weight control had not progressed much beyond my mother's store of folk wisdom. The key to lasting weight loss had eluded all of them. I was disappointed. I had expected more from these men who had spent their careers researching the condition of obesity.

In fact, this feeling had crept into a number of peoples' heads around that time. The absence of effective treatments for excess weight helped launch the antidiet movement that was gaining force even as these scientists gathered. People like Susan Powter, the fitness guru whose late-night infomercials exhorted us to "Stop the Insanity!" had already begun to ride the nationwide wave of frustration. Others more quietly threw up their hands in disgust, and the McLean disappeared off McDonald's menu, making way for the Arch Deluxe with bacon.

But by the end of the conference I felt that my initial reaction had been too hasty. Though these scientists had not yet figured out how to help people reliably lose weight, their talks outlined a new way of looking at the issue. They showed where the real research progress was being made—

not in sure-fire diet strategies, but in understanding the molecular and genetic basis of weight. I began to see that over the last decade these scientists had been sowing a rich field, pursuing the genes, proteins, and neurochemicals that govern eating and energy use. And late the following year, one of those seeds produced a magnificent flower.

On December 1, 1994, scientists at Rockefeller University in New York announced their discovery of the *obese* gene in mice. Some newspaper articles mistakenly described it as *the* obesity gene. Early results hinted that it might be *the* key to what makes us get fat. The ensuing years have shown the genetics of obesity to be much richer and more complicated than that. Nonetheless, the *obese* gene remains a landmark discovery, not least because of its triumph over stereotypes. Virtually overnight, it introduced millions of people to the idea that overweight was not a personality defect. You don't have to be a sloth or a glutton to be fat. The *obese* discovery substantiated what many had long suspected—that weight problems lurk in some peoples' DNA.

As the talks at that early obesity seminar suggested, the *obese* gene was merely the opening salvo of a barrage of genetic and biological discoveries in the years that followed. Hard science has finally begun to take the problem of weight control seriously. The molecular approach to studying weight is already offering insights into why diets don't work and new possibilities for weight control that will involve getting in and tinkering with our bodies on the level of proteins and neurotransmitters. As a result of such efforts, scientists are gradually stumbling toward a new definition of fat—one that is more mechanistic and less freighted with guilt.

That definition extends well beyond the nuts and bolts of genes and proteins. Roles are played by the fatty food we eat and the exercise we don't get, by a high-stress culture and an obsession with thinness that warps our relationship with food. The media deserve some of the blame for encouraging this obsession. Television shoulders even more responsibility for our sedentary ways. Boredom, unhappiness, and ignorance all play an undeniable role in our slide up the scale. But so does biology. In the search to understand what causes us to gain weight, the sheer force of our own physiology has too often been given short shrift.

One of the goals of this book is to give readers a way of thinking about their bodies they may not have considered before—a more scientific way of seeing things. In doing so, I have also tried to shed some light on what happens when the scientific view of obesity collides with the nitty-gritty world of life outside the lab. Here in the land of plenty, where bathroom scales abound and mayonnaise is a battleground, any effort to make sense of obesity research requires that we see it through the eyes of those who struggle with its findings.

It will come as no surprise, therefore, that this is a book of extremes. The voices in it range from biologists who tinker with the chemical messengers of obesity to the fat activists who call these scientists pigs, from the fat phobic who exert militaristic control over their bodies to those who have placed authority over their weight in the hands of a higher being. Some of these examples may strike readers as laughable, others as too familiar. In one way or another they illuminate the strange and complex ways that research on fat has worked its way into our daily lives.

I would like to make it clear that you don't have to consider yourself obese to get something out of this book. Obesity may not be what you think it is. "Obese" is one of those words that means one thing to a layman's ear and another thing to a scientist. Ask the average person to define obese and they will spread their arms wide enough to span a 60-inch waistline. Scientists refer to people in this weight category as morbidly obese.

Scientifically, the word obese describes anyone who weighs at least 24 percent more than their medically ideal weight, and a lot of us do. A quarter of Americans are obese, according to the latest health surveys. That figure jumped from a steady 14 percent of the population throughout the 1960s and 1970s, and the rapid upward trend is expected to continue. Recently John Foreyt, an obesity researcher at the Baylor College of Medicine in Houston, calculated that the United States is heading toward 100 percent obesity by the year 2230. While the rates in most other westernized nations aren't nearly as high, they are rising in many places at the same rapid clip.

Whether or not you qualify as obese under this scientific definition, the point I would like to emphasize is that what goes for those on the heavy end of the scale goes for those at the light end, too. As this book explains in more detail, we are all part of a continuum of people who are more or less susceptible to obesity. There is no line in the sand between people who are obese and people who are overweight, or for that matter people who don't worry about their weight. This book, and the research it describes, are about health and weight regulation in all people.

You may be reading this book because you're tired of the confusing bombardment of information and want to know how much of it is believable. You may be struggling with weight or are just interested in the latest discoveries. You may have read about the *obese* gene but aren't really sure how it affects you. Doesn't the latest genetic research on obesity imply that we're pretty much going to end up shaped like our mothers or fathers no matter what we do? If that's the case, then why do so many health experts persist in telling us that we should eat less fat? Isn't it true that diets don't work? Isn't there an easier way to lose weight?

Perhaps you heard about the diet drugs that were yanked off the market a few years ago for dangerous side effects. But you may not realize that there is a host of new ones coming to take their place. Are they safe? Do they work? Will there ever be a pill that will let us eat what we want without getting fat? Answering such questions is largely what this book is about.

The book doesn't promise a miracle program for weight loss. It won't put you in a "zone." But once you finish reading it, you will know what specialists in the field think about why we gain weight, and you'll know what tools are available to help you get to your own weight goal. You will also understand your own body much better, which will be a great asset in helping you work with your weight-control system instead of against it.

Much of the health research that is reported in newspapers and magazines comes out of the field of epidemiology, a branch of science that studies disease on a population-wide basis. Particularly influential have been the prospective studies, like the Nurses Health Study and the Framingham Heart Study, that follow large groups of people over many years to see how different behaviors impact health. While researching this book I sat in on a group of mostly epidemiologists that meets biweekly at the Harvard School of Public Health to talk about such research in nutrition and obesity. As enlightening as those group meetings were, I can't help but feel that the epidemiological studies on weight are the source of much of our current confusion. Partly that is a result of the fact that the media is so quick to publicize any weight-related research. Contradictory results, which are the essence of any scientific pursuit, leave people not knowing which information to believe. Partly it is because epidemiology, as a way of understanding obesity, goes only so far.

Good epidemiologists know that when they find a link between any aspect of human behavior and a health problem, it becomes meaningful only if they can provide a plausible biological mechanism that shows how the cause relates to the effect. For something like the relationship between cigarette smoking and lung cancer, epidemiologists don't have to work too hard to convince most people that there is a plausible mechanism. But when it comes to studies linking overweight and mortality, it's difficult for epidemiologists to say whether obese people suffer more health risks because of their weight or simply because their weight prevents them from exercising. In the end, I found that much of the epidemiological research wasn't addressing the kinds of questions I wanted answered, and therefore I have tended in this book to leap over it and head straight for the mechanisms.

How much of our body shape we inherit and how much we bring on ourselves seems to be one of the most basic issues when it comes to weight. So this is where the book begins—first with a look at what it means, both physically and culturally, when people say that fat is in our genes. Chapter Two then describes some background on the curious road we have taken to get to the *obese* gene discovery. The story of a plump little mouse is part of a much larger history of what has happened when our culture has adopted and adapted scientific research on how to control weight.

I don't think I'll be giving too much away by telling you that genes don't explain everything. There is an undeniable measure of personal control in what happens to our bodies. How, then, are people supposed to maintain healthy weights? With high-protein regimes, say the diet gurus. With vigorous exercise, say the fitness experts. Maybe just moderate exercise, says the Center for Disease Control and Prevention, in an effort to encourage the sedentary masses to do something, anything, rather than sit on the sofa night after night. Chapters Three and Four look at efforts to exert conscious control over our weight through diet and exercise and what the latest scientific research says about how our bodies respond.

Peppered throughout the conversations of doctors and obesity researchers are references to the idea that obesity is a disease—a chronic illness that demands chronic treatment, a public health threat that costs our nation nearly $100 billion a year. One of the effects of this medicalization of obesity is a new attitude toward drug treatment. Over the next decade we will be seeing an avalanche of new diet drugs. Pharmaceutical companies that avoided them for many years have now leapt into development, and the FDA is struggling to deal with this new approach to treatment.

Chapter Five looks at weight-control drugs from different angles. On the one hand, the mix of diet drugs and our culture has already produced disastrous results. People have tried the newest versions of these drugs in droves without regard for how the drugs are meant to work. On the other hand, the pieces of the body's weight-control machinery are beginning to come together for researchers like the cogs of a Swiss watch. The drugs that these molecular insights produce may bring precision, power, and extraordinary relief to people who struggle with their weight.

The same people have understandably mixed reactions to the news that their looks are a disease that needs to be cured. Even as scientific research has lifted some of the burden of shame from obese people, the medical war against the condition has escalated. Chapter Six takes a deeper look at this situation. Some size activists, seeing little to distinguish social concern about the health risks of obesity from age-old bigotry, are waging war against fat phobia instead. Others are searching gamely for a middle ground, where the efforts of doctors, researchers, and drug manufacturers address the true health needs of the obese population.

The fact that people get fat for different reasons is one of the most helpful insights to come out of obesity research in the last decade. We may all have the same basic equipment, but that doesn't diminish the multitude of differences in how our bodies control weight. The result of this insight is that weight control of the future may be individualized. Part of our maturation in understanding weight will be not only accepting that bodies handle food and exercise in different ways, but in gaining the tools to define and measure the differences and to help people chart their own weight course using the results. Chapter Seven proposes a future scenario for our scientific understanding of weight.

For now the mantra among many obesity specialists is prevention of weight gain. Achieving a stable weight, though far from easy, is the healthiest course for all weight classes. Chapter Eight discusses what people can do now in terms of applying, both to their own lives and to those of their children, what scientists have learned about weight to lead healthy lives.

Whether we are fat or not, we are all part of the effort to get a handle on our bodies and on what constitutes healthy living. Science is one lens through which we can look. In doing so, we can begin to see what elements in our culture and in our nature are likely to undermine the products of weight research, and we can begin to ask whether science can reverse the current trend toward escalating obesity. On a fundamental level, the question of whether or not a more biological way of looking at fat will help people come to grips with their bodies is bigger than the science itself. It has to encompass the weight-conscious culture in which these discoveries are made. The story of how we as a society are searching for the roots of our obesity in research labs at the same time that we as individuals desperately try to get our weight under control is the story of the human condition—the universal struggle against our own nature as we struggle to understand it. This book represents a slice of that rich pie.

ONE

All in the Family

ARE WE GENETICALLY
PROGRAMMED
TO BE FAT?

John Rossi had worked at the Kragen Auto Parts store in Berkeley, California for ten consecutive years, first as a clerk and then as a manager. He was a model employee, missing only three days in all that time and regularly working 50- to 60-hour weeks. So it was something of a surprise when one July day, Rossi's manager told him not to come into work anymore.

A spokesman for the store later said that Rossi was fired for poor job performance. But the only reason Rossi could see for his dismissal was the fact that he was fat. A high school football star, Rossi had struggled with obesity throughout his adult life. He had seen his weight soar to 275 pounds by the age of 21, when he first started working at Kragen. And over the next decade he tried everything, from fasting to hypnosis. He even wired his jaws shut. But in spite of his efforts, Rossi's weight continued to climb. On the day he was fired he weighed about 400 pounds.

The weight encumbers Rossi. It is difficult for him to sit, stand, and walk. But it never affected his job performance, as shown by the company's own evaluations along with laudatory letters from customers. Therefore Rossi did what any self-respecting person would do under the circumstances. He sued.

His case, brought under the California Fair Employment and Housing Act, became a landmark in our societal definition of what it means to be fat, though it was by no means the first such suit to test the way the courts treat the overweight. Under the same law, a Santa Cruz woman named Toni Cassista filed a discrimination suit against Community Foods, Inc., a health food store that refused to hire her because of her severe obesity.

Cassista's case did not go well. In 1993, the California supreme court ruled against her. The court decided that employment discrimination against an obese person wasn't illegal unless it could be proved that the person's weight was the result of a physiological disorder. In other words, the courts treated Cassista's obesity as a condition that she could change if only she set her mind to it.

That ruling was in line with popular assumptions about obesity—that it is caused by a lack of willpower; that people who become obese simply need to push themselves away from the table sooner. And if that were truly the case, it would have been very much in agreement with the way disability law is intended to work. In most states it is perfectly legal to fire someone if you think they are ugly or smell bad and you don't want to put up with them any longer. Only if they have a physical or mental impairment—a condition beyond their control—are they protected by the Americans with Disabilities Act and similar laws in many states.

Cassista, though she clearly felt she was being discriminated against because of an involuntary condition, never saw her weight as a disability. She therefore felt that it would be unconscionable to claim such a thing in court. The result of her principled stance was that her lawyer never called on an expert witness to explain the medical basis of her weight, and Cassista lost the case.

Lynette Labinger was loath to make the same mistake. Two days after the Cassista decision came down, Labinger, an attorney, was scheduled to argue a similar case—the appeal of Bonnie Cook. Cook sued the state of Rhode Island for refusing to hire her at a home for retarded people. She had worked at the home before, from 1978 to 1980 and again from 1981 to 1986. Both times she had left voluntarily, and with a clean employment record. But in 1988, when she applied for the job a third time, she weighed more than 320 pounds—significantly more than she had during her prior years of employment at the home. The physician responsible for approving her application rejected it, claiming that her weight compromised her ability to evacuate patients in an emergency and increased her risk for heart disease, thereby increasing the likelihood that she would need worker's compensation.

The fact that the Cassista decision was negative sounded an ominous warning for Cook and certainly would have influenced Labinger's tactics had it come a little earlier. As it was, Labinger didn't have a lot of time to dwell on the implications of the ruling. "I was scrambling around, reading the decision, trying to figure out how I was going to deal with it in oral argument," she says.

Fortunately, she had done her homework. As part of the preparation for the jury trial she lined up Arthur Frank, Medical Director for the Obesity Management Program at the George Washington University School of Medicine in Washington, D.C., as an expert medical witness. Trained in biochemistry but with a psychological bent, Frank is an individual of overwhelming humanity. He gracefully straddles the awkward boundary between the biochemical underpinnings of obesity and the very human task of coping with it daily.

He began his testimony by dispelling the myth that people have a lot of say about their weight. Using himself as an example, he told the jury that he was "a random eater. I don't pay any attention to what I eat and over the last twenty years my weight hasn't changed at all." Then, to paint a mental picture, he explained that the number of calories he would have to eat in order to put on an extra pound a year amounted to no more than a few peanuts a day. Knowing that to be the case, he said, any reasonable person would have to conclude that our bodies take care of our weight without any conscious help.

"Nature does not permit body weight to fluctuate randomly in other mammals," Frank wrote in a commentary published around the time that he appeared in court. "It is inconceivable that humans would have a randomly unstable weight. Even obese people are usually weight stable, albeit at an inappropriate level. We weigh what we are supposed to weigh, and the regulatory systems defend that weight with remarkable physiologic tenacity." Although Frank made it clear in this commentary that people can at times override these controls by deliberate effort or because their emotional climate changes, he wrote, "There is no reason to believe that patients' behavior causes this disease."

Frank wasn't saying that people couldn't gain weight by overeating—just that it is difficult to fatten people up unless their bodies are susceptible to it. He also wasn't saying that obesity couldn't be an outgrowth of a psychological trauma like childhood abuse. But in his eyes, psychology has little to do with causing people to overeat or to be fat. Rather, he says, it plays a role in their ability to cope with gaining weight and their comfort in sustaining a heavy weight once they've reached it.

Frank's straightforward view of obesity sliced through the stereotypes. People so often blame emotions for excess weight. They think there is something psychologically wrong with people that causes them to be fat. As a result, fat people have guilt heaped on them by society, in addition to the physical burden they themselves carry. But in Frank's comments to the jury, he maintained that there were clear biochemical reasons why people crave something sweet at a certain hour of the day or a bowlful of pasta when they are feeling stressed, and the reasons have nothing whatsoever to do with will power.

Frank took the wind out of the sails of anyone in the courtroom who assumed that if obese people would just eat better and exercise more they wouldn't look the way they do. His testimony meant that for someone like Cook, the requirement that she lose weight to get a job was the equivalent of a sentence to starve herself. She might be able to do it, but the biological drive to eat would linger as long as the weight was gone.

The jury took Frank's words to heart. Cook won her case and its subsequent appeal, setting a precedent in the federal court system. Two years later, John Rossi's jury also granted him a victory. The verdict established a separate precedent in the California courts, but it was the size of the award that made this case a landmark. Rossi's jury granted him the sum of $1,035,652 for lost compensation and emotional distress.

When Rossi heard the verdict in the courtroom, he finally let out his tears. After a four-year battle of legal depositions, settlement meetings, and testimony, he was finally the hero of the story instead of the victim. The million-dollar verdict put the final nail in the coffin of obesity discrimination lawsuits. And just as in the Cook case, what had convinced Rossi's jury was the science.

The key to the verdict, according to Rossi's lawyer, Barbara Lawless, was testimony by an expert medical witness that obesity is 80 percent genetic. Actually, the 80 percent figure is at the high end of the range usually given by experts in the genetics of obesity. Most researchers' estimates hover around 50 percent. But there is an overwhelming store of evidence pointing to the fact that weight is at least 5 percent and in some cases as much as 90 percent inherited. Where the courts have based their decisions on this scientific research, weight discrimination suits have triumphed.

Yet the legal travails of Rossi and Cook bring up an important point. The courts protected them from discrimination because they could make a clear case that their morbid obesity was an immutable condition. In doing so, however, the courts have drawn a sharp cutoff where in biology only a blurry boundary exists.

There is no magic line between being morbidly obese (which is defined as body weight more than 100 percent above the norm) and being merely overweight. Genetic research shows that they are just different aspects of a continuum that extends all the way down the weight scale from the minority of people who weigh upwards of 300 pounds to the vast majority who would just like to lose the spare tire they have gained since high school. All these people simply have a greater or lesser genetic susceptibility to gaining weight.

That's where things get confusing. Susceptibility? The word doesn't fit neatly into what we know about nature or nurture. It doesn't spell out a clear path for what people should do to lose weight. And yet, the genetic roots of this susceptibility are key to the rise in weight in this country. They dictate the extent to which any of us is destined to cling to that extra 20 pounds. They explain why two people can eat exactly the same amount and only one of them will get fat. As a result, genetics has taken on great importance for scientists trying to understand why people get fat.

Inheriting Fat

For over 20 years, families of French descent living within 50 miles of Quebec city have been voluntarily subjecting themselves to a battery of tests in order to help researchers understand how genes affect our weight. Paul-André Sauvageau, a retired civil engineer, and his family were among the first to join the Quebec Family Study. In 1979, Sauvageau took his wife, his 12-year-old son, and 10-year-old daughter to the Physical Activity Sciences Laboratory at Laval University in Ste-Foy. He was 47 at the time and an avid skier. His wife, a dietitian, was ten years younger.

Like Olympic decathloners, the family members took turns at half a dozen testing stations. They skipped their usual breakfast so that the technicians could measure their energy use in the fasting state and then again after they ate. They rode a stationary bicycle while doctors and technicians kept an eye on their heartbeats and other vital signs. They gave blood for what seemed to Sauvageau like a very long time. They strapped on weights and were plunged into the underwater weighing tank.

Sauvageau's wife didn't enjoy that test much. Nor did his sister-in-law, who also went to the lab along with three of Sauvageau's brothers-in-law and their children. But the extended family went back in 1991 and did the tests over again for phase 2 of the study, which looked at a subset of the original families. The Quebec Family Study data set now extends from 1978 to the present, and both because of this length and because of the thoroughness of the testing, it constitutes one of the best scientific resources on the genetics of health.

The study is the brainchild of a soft-spoken and highly regarded geneticist at Laval named Claude Bouchard. From the beginning Bouchard's plan was to look at the effect of genetic and nongenetic factors on body composition, on the response to exercise, on muscular strength, and on standard blood measurements, like pressure, cholesterol and fat content. But over the years the obesity component of the study has become by far the most prominent, perhaps because in the last two decades the weights of Canadians have increased just as quickly as those of Americans. A third of the populations of both countries are now obese. "Yeah," Bouchard says with a wry smile, "we share so many things."

Of course, finding the genetic component of obesity is slightly different from saying that it is something you get from your parents. Things like eating habits and attitudes toward food can be passed down simply because family members eat, sleep, and breathe under the same roof, which is why for many years it was difficult to say just how strong a role genes play in our eating behavior.

But studies during the mid-1980s of identical twins helped tease apart the roles played in obesity by family environment and genes. Nowadays, nearly everyone is familiar with the stories of twins who have been separated for decades and then, when they finally reunite, can't help noticing an extraordinary number of similarities in the way they do everything from zip their pants to choose careers. This phenomenon also applies to BMI, or body mass index, a measure of weight in kilograms relative to height in meters (see the chart on the following page). Studies comparing identical twins reared apart with twins reared together show that biology is a much stronger influence on weight than family environment. The best estimates from twin studies say that between 40 and 70 percent of our BMI is determined by our genes.

Weight (lbs.) Height	100	105	110	115	120	125	130	135	140	145	150	155	160	165	170	175	180	185	190	195	200	205	210	215	220	225	230	235	240	245	250
5'0"	20	21	21	22	23	24	25	26	27	28	29	30	31	32	33	34	35	36	37	38	39	40	41	42	43	44	45	46	47	48	49
5'1"	19	20	21	22	23	24	24	25	26	27	28	29	30	31	32	33	34	35	36	37	38	39	40	41	42	43	44	44	45	46	47
5'2"	18	19	20	21	22	23	24	25	26	27	27	28	29	30	31	32	33	34	35	36	37	37	38	39	40	41	42	43	44	45	46
5'3"	18	19	19	20	21	22	23	24	25	26	27	27	28	29	30	31	32	33	34	35	35	36	37	38	39	40	41	42	43	43	44
5'4"	17	18	19	20	21	21	22	23	24	25	26	27	27	28	29	30	31	32	33	33	34	35	36	37	38	39	39	40	41	42	43
5'5"	17	17	18	19	20	21	22	22	23	24	25	26	27	27	28	29	30	31	32	32	33	34	35	36	37	37	38	39	40	41	42
5'6"	16	17	18	19	19	20	21	22	23	23	24	25	26	27	27	28	29	30	31	31	32	33	34	35	36	36	37	38	39	40	40
5'7"	16	16	17	18	19	20	20	21	22	23	23	24	25	26	27	27	28	29	30	31	31	32	33	34	34	35	36	37	38	38	39
5'8"	15	16	17	17	18	19	20	21	21	22	23	24	24	25	26	27	27	28	29	30	30	31	32	33	33	34	35	36	36	37	38
5'9"	15	16	16	17	18	18	19	20	21	21	22	23	24	24	25	26	27	27	28	29	30	30	31	32	32	33	34	35	35	36	37
5'10"	14	15	16	16	17	18	19	19	20	21	22	22	23	24	24	25	26	27	27	28	29	29	30	31	32	32	33	34	34	35	36
5'11"	14	15	15	16	17	17	18	19	20	20	21	22	22	23	24	24	25	26	26	27	28	29	29	30	31	31	32	33	33	34	35
6'0"	14	14	15	16	16	17	18	18	19	20	20	21	22	22	23	24	24	25	26	26	27	28	28	29	30	31	31	32	33	33	34
6'1"	13	14	15	15	16	16	17	18	18	19	20	20	21	22	22	23	24	24	25	26	26	27	28	28	29	30	30	31	32	32	33
6'2"	13	13	14	15	15	16	17	17	18	19	19	20	21	21	22	22	23	24	24	25	26	26	27	28	28	29	30	30	31	31	32
6'3"	12	13	14	14	15	16	16	17	17	18	19	19	20	21	21	22	22	23	24	24	25	26	26	27	27	28	29	29	30	31	31
6'4"	12	13	13	14	15	15	16	16	17	18	18	19	19	20	21	21	22	23	23	24	24	25	26	26	27	27	28	29	29	30	30

Body mass index chart. Researchers prefer to use body mass index, or BMI, to assess a person's level of fatness because the measurement incorporates both height and weight. A BMI of 30 or more is the clinical definition of obese.

In recent years, Bouchard's group has used their extensive data set to build on the estimates and show that not only BMI but a broad range of weight traits are hereditary. Bouchard and his colleagues have amassed information on body fat, on insulin metabolism, on fat within the bloodstream, on resting metabolic rate. They have done CT scans to measure visceral fat—fat that is located around internal organs like the heart, liver, or intestines. And they have collected cell lines for each family member, providing them access to each individual's DNA.

They have shown that one of the most important aspects of weight maintenance, our resting metabolic rate, or how much energy we burn when we aren't being active, is largely determined by our genes. Resting metabolism accounts for about 70 percent of the energy, or food, we burn in a given day. And studies by Bouchard's group as well as others suggest that 40 to 80 percent of the variance in this resting rate is inherited.

That doesn't necessarily mean that our DNA dictates whether we are one of those people who juggle sixteen projects simultaneously or among those who live by the tortoise's decree: slow and steady wins the race. People assume that metabolism is the key to how much vigor people have. But Bouchard's group has shown that genes exert only a small influence on how much general activity we do in a day. That means not just exercise but all kinds of activities. The researchers attribute only about 29 percent of the variation in this trait to genes. While active parents do indeed give rise to active children, it is mostly because they socialize their children to be that way.

There is also a genetic component to whether you will get a swag of loose flesh on your upper arm as you age or whether your ankles will stay sleek in spite of a bulging middle. In other words, genes affect not only whether you are fat but also where you are fat. Whether you have the shape of an apple or a pear has important consequences for how detrimental the extra weight you're carrying is to your health. Fat around our bellies is associated with a greater risk of diabetes, heart disease and hypertension, whereas hip and thigh fat is relatively benign. It may be easier to hide a bulging middle under a baggy sweater, but for health reasons a pear shape is good, an apple shape is bad. Heredity accounts for as much as 40 percent of the variance in the distribution of fat.

To a lesser extent, genes also influence how much fat is stored when we eat excess food. Overindulge, and your genes will show you whether you are one of those people who turn excess food into fat very efficiently or if you are a relative failure at fatmaking. Genes also determine how effective an exercise program will be in helping you lose weight. Dedicate yourself to daily exercise, and your genes will decide whether your commitment will lead to massive weight loss or a paltry few pounds.

There is also a genetic component to the kinds of food we decide to eat. Many people have already caught on to their own food preferences. They know they will pass up a bowl of candy for a juicy steak any day. Research has shown that steak lovers tend to beget steak lovers; roughly 10 to 20 percent of food selection is under genetic control.

Perhaps none of this is surprising. When we grow up we end up looking and acting a lot like our parents. It doesn't take a genius to realize that weight problems run in families. The apple doesn't fall far from the tree. But most of us also carry the notion that socialization has a large role in familial similarity. Your mother may have made an extraordinary plate of spaghetti in her day, and it's easy to assume that your current love of pasta is the result of that culinary tradition.

Many of us also feel that we have a large measure of choice as to whether we follow our parents' patterns. So it is interesting to learn to what extent not only our looks but our habits are hard-wired. Perhaps your mother spent so much time perfecting her spaghetti recipe because somewhere deep within her DNA was a carbohydrate-craving gene.

The fact that genes influence weight, however, doesn't mean that they are entirely to blame for the expansion of our nation's waistlines. The unspoken message in all these genetic percentages is that they are just that—percentages. Fractions. Our weight isn't 100 percent inherited. Indeed, a great deal of cultural evidence indicates that weight is partly the product of environment, a term researchers use to mean things like the food choices that are available, as well as how sedentary people are or how often they eat out.

Jose Caro, an obesity specialist at Lilly Research Labs in Indianapolis, once illustrated the impact of environment by describing his impressions from a trip to Beijing. "It's incredible what you see," he said. "The adult Chinese are elegant looking, thin. They eat rice and they ride bicycles. They are allowed to have only one child, and almost 100 percent of the children are obese. So you see you have a very weird situation where you have the overlap at the same time of a lean environment and an obese environment. The parents believe that what they were doing was bad and they were suffering and now they want to compensate and give more to their only child. So they take them to McDonalds. They don't allow their child to ride the bicycle; they buy electric motors. And you see these genes haven't changed." While the genetic heritage of these children remains the same, the environment in which they are reared allows for an alarming increase in obesity.

Caro's Chinese example may be anecdotal, but sudden leaps in the rate of obesity are common whenever people go from one food environment to another. Charles Rotimi, an obesity researcher at the Loyola University Medical Center, studied this phenomenon in his adopted town of Chicago. He found that when men and women from his former homeland, Nigeria, as well as Cameroon, emigrate to the land of the deep-dish pizza, their obesity rates skyrocket.

The average rural African Rotimi looked at had a body mass index of about 21, which means that a 6-foot man weighed about 155 pounds. By contrast, the average African who had moved to Chicago had a BMI of 30, which translates into a weight of 220 pounds for a man of the same height. African émigrés in the Caribbean and in Manchester, England, fell between these two extremes. "Basically it was just a very steep gradient from rural Africa through the Caribbean islands to Chicago," says Rotimi.

"The assumption here, of course, is that these are populations of similar heritage in vastly different environments."

Rotimi has also found a lesser but still significant jump in the obesity rates when Nigerians move from rural areas to African cities."The urban poor in Nigeria, which is the majority of the population, are struggling to meet daily nutritional requirements," he says. "But even within these sub-Saharan countries, if you look at the urban elite, they have this problem of obesity."

In the affluent West, the problem is even more severe and has grown worse over the last decade. The incidence of obesity in the United States had held steady at about 14 percent of the population since 1960, when the government began its National Health and Nutrition Examination Surveys. Then, between 1981 and 1991, it shot up to a quarter of Americans. This is on top of the gradual rise in the prevalence of obesity that has taken place over the last century. Both these increases have occurred far too quickly to be attributed to a change in our population's genetic makeup.

What's happening is that our existing genes are conspiring with our evolving environment to make us fat. "You start with some people who are more at risk," explains University of Pennsylvania geneticist Arlen Price, "and you make high-fat diets available to everyone and everyone gains weight and some people in particular really gain a lot. So you can actually see the gene-environment interactions changing in real time over the last century."

America's rising rate of obesity has been accompanied by shifts in who is affected. Twenty to thirty years ago it was more the norm for a prosperous person to be over-weight—a "fat cat." The prevalence of obesity was sub-stantially higher in upper-income groups than it is today. Now being overweight is no longer a status symbol. In addition, the better educated you are and the higher your income, the less likely you are to be sedentary, a radical shift in behavior within the population. In contrast with the time when vigorous activity was generally associated with lower socioeconomic status—literally the working class—physical activity has now become a luxury. Yet the fact that wealthy, educated groups have managed to control obesity indicates how strong an influence lifestyle can be.

Genes may not be everything, but compared to the tan-gled social fabric of fast-food meals, cities with no walking paths, and the American love affair with cars, genes are something scientists can locate, identify and isolate for careful scrutiny. And in the pursuit of obesity's genetic roots, what is ultimately important is not the percentage of body shape or metabolic rate that we inherit, but what spe-cific genes affect weight and what variations in them cause weight to balloon. For while genes may not be wholly responsible for the way we look, they can have an enor-mous impact on some people. In the cutthroat arena of body consciousness, just where you fit on the continuum of nature versus nurture is critically important.

Susceptibility and Resistance

"Some people have the good genes, some people don't," says geneticist David West with a kind of John Wayne bluntness. West is seated in his office at the Pennington Biomedical Research Center in Baton Rouge, Louisiana. He is telling me that for a minority of obese people, their genes are their body's destiny. "I think there are some patients," he says, "especially the very morbidly obese patient, who are going to be pretty much a biological problem. They have a real nasty set of genes. As long as they have enough calories to eat they're going to be fat no matter what environment they're in and despite their best efforts."

These are people like Rossi, Cassista, and Cook, who have led the fight to have that fact acknowledged. But whereas one can make a clear case that biology pretty much rules at the high end of the continuum, farther down, where the genetic susceptibility to gaining weight is only moderate, it also takes a certain lifestyle to push weight skyward. West, who counts himself among the vast sea of people who are "a little overweight," says that in order for people like him to size up, they have to do things like sit behind a desk all day, wolf down a big lunch, collapse at home in the evening with a few beers, and then wake up the next morning to repeat it all again. They might also want to hold down a stressful job, take on a little too much responsibility at home, or just get in the habit of watching too much television.

Can do.

In a nutshell, what's causing most of us to hold onto a few extra pounds each year—pounds that don't go away even at the summer's end—is how our genes interact with our environment. Our genes make us susceptible to obesity, and the habits of being sedentary and overindulging push us over the edge.

In a way, we are a lot like a group of mice that West has been studying for more than a decade. The mice are normal rodents that get fat only when they are fed a particularly delectable brand of rat chow. High in fat and sugar, the chow most resembles chocolate chip cookie dough without the chips—just sugar, shortening and powdered rodent food.

Researchers call the animals that succumb to such meals DIO, or diet-induced obesity, mice. There is also a group of DIO mice that become obese only when they are offered many different and tasty items simultaneously. This diet is known in the trade as a "supermarket" or "cafeteria" diet, and its similarity to the kind of food available to most people needs no elaboration beyond these names.

When DIO mice become fat they show all the associated biological changes people show. Their blood pressure and blood sugar go up, their metabolic rate increases, and their circulating insulin levels rise even as they become insulin resistant. The genetic roots of their weight gain also parallel those in people. They have many genes that make them susceptible to weight gain when they are put in a certain environment—one with calorie-dense, highly palatable foods.

Researchers believe that people have a similar genetic profile. They think that many genes contribute to what we weigh, just as many genes contribute to how tall we become. These are genes that guide a tiny embryo through the stages of creating a brand new set of organs as well as genes that kick in at puberty or later in life. Rather than making us inevitably, unalterably fat, these genes make us more susceptible to weight gain. And that susceptibility may only kick in when we encounter the right surroundings—the kind of place where Big Macs and Ding-Dongs are available around the clock and only a short car ride away.

But just as genes can make us susceptible to obesity, they can also make us resistant. One thing that's particularly intriguing about the DIO mice is that in some strains a few of the animals do not become obese in spite of efforts to fatten them up. All the animals are fed the same diet, and while 75 percent of them become obese, a quarter of them don't. This means researchers have within their grasp not only mice that are susceptible to diet-induced obesity, but also mice that are resistant to it. Something allows these animals to stay skinny even as their littermates succumb to a junky diet.

West thinks that individual mice or mouse strains that are resistant to dietary obesity have metabolic adaptations that limit the amount of body fat they can accumulate. "So if you put them on a high fat diet," he says, "they are, for example, very effective at increasing metabolic rate to compensate for the additional calories" or at adjusting their fat cells in a way that makes them less efficient at storing fat.

Just how those alterations are played out in the body is still an open question, but by studying the genetic variations between the obesity-resistant and obesity-susceptible strains, it should be possible to find the answer. From there it is a short jump to ask why some people can eat more than other people and never gain weight—the question Richard Surwit, an obesity researcher at Duke University Medical Center in Durham, North Carolina, says "is really what everybody's interested in."

"You've got to have an explanation," he says, "for why there are certain individuals who are skin and bones and can eat all the fat they want. I think that's where the secret to obesity is. I think it's not in obese people, it's in lean people. Why are certain people able to eat what they want with impunity?"

The obesity-resistant mice then, are the waif models of the mouse community—anomalies of nature, if you will, like albino alligators or six-toed cats, which drive home the point that just as some people are prone to obesity, others are virtually immune to it. Researchers can comb through the DNA of the resistant mice and find out how it differs from that of the susceptible mice. And really we are talking here about the search for flipsides of the same coin—obesity-resistant genes that are slight variations of obesity-susceptible genes. If you have a certain version you're more likely to get fat, and if you have a different sequence you are less likely to get fat. Researchers can then use the genes that make mice susceptible or resistant to obesity to search for the same sorts of genes in people.

Interestingly, the same idea of genetic resistance and susceptibility applies not only to obesity but to obesity-related illnesses. West says, "There are a fair number of people walking around out there who are 60, 80 pounds overweight and, you know, have normal blood sugar, normal blood pressure. Their joints are fine. They don't have gall bladder disease. There doesn't seem to be a greater risk for cancer. Why? I think it's because they have another set of genes that protects them from these adverse effects of being fat."

A group of researchers at Rockefeller University who are working on the question of illness susceptibility are finding that some obese strains of mice get diabetes, others do not. By mapping the genes that confer susceptibility and resistance, the group is looking for answers to a different but related set of questions. What is it that allows some overweight people to stay healthy while others become ill?

Such research is helping us move beyond the percentages of many genetic studies to the genes that are making us obese in the current environment. Researchers can find the susceptibility and resistance genes first in mice where it is easier, quicker, and cheaper to do research. Then they can determine whether the analogous regions on the human DNA chain are also linked to obesity or its related diseases. And DIO mice are thought to be better candidates for helping researchers find what makes the average person gain weight.

The conviction among scientists that most people have not one but many genes contributing to their weight implies that the genes that make DIO mice susceptible to obesity are more likely to have echoes in the human population. Recently Bouchard and his colleagues used their extensive list of families to link one such DIO gene with a region on the human DNA chain. Dozens of similar obesity gene candidates are likewise stacking up as a result of collaborative work between other research groups who collect families and those who comb through mouse DNA. Though the exact genes still await discovery, the research paints a vivid picture of where the field is headed. Human genes for susceptibility to obesity are likely to be found in the coming years. Biologists will then be able to figure out what these genes and the proteins they produce do inside our bodies.

Inevitably some of these genes and proteins will be found to have greater effects on our weight than others. So while some researchers are plowing forward with the arduous task of identifying the many genes that contribute to weight gain, others like Bouchard are working on a parallel track. They are trying to focus the effort on the genes that affect the largest number of people.

Major Genes

Over the last ten years Bouchard and his collaborators at the Washington University School of Medicine in St. Louis have amassed evidence from their statistical analyses of the Quebec data that a few of key genes lie within the mixed bag of obesity-related DNA. These key, or major, genes have large effects, as opposed to the small cumulative effects that most human obesity genes have. Thus they are likely to be the main causes of weight gain for the bulk of the population.

Bouchard's team has found that a major gene is responsible for the amount of fat we carry on our bodies.

There is also a major gene for the ratio of trunk fat to limb fat, although at the moment the researchers don't know whether the major genes for these two traits are actually one and the same. They have strong evidence, however, for a distinct major gene for what biologists call deep visceral fat. This is the fat that resides in our abdominal cavity. Some studies have shown that it may be slightly easier to lose this fat than the fat on our hips and thighs. It is also what gives people an apple shape, thus making it the most dangerous fat in the human body.

Another distinct major gene affects resting metabolic rate. Bouchard's group estimates that a subgroup of individuals—about 7 percent of the population—seems to be well endowed to resist weight gain because they are genetically predisposed to possess a high metabolism. The rest of us are either neutral or more susceptible to obesity because of lower metabolic rates. Such results may be depressing, but they are also good news in the sense that they imply that we may one day understand the biological causes of obesity for large numbers of people. As we learn more about the main genes responsible for weight gain, we can ask what aspects of our environment have the biggest effects on those genes.

The existence of major genes also raises the possibility that drugs may be developed that will be broadly effective. The implications of such drugs and how they might work is grist for Chapter Five. Lest we get ahead of ourselves, it will be some time before the impacts of this genetic research are felt. In the meantime, the knowledge that weight is only partially attributable to our genes leaves no doubt that for at least some of us who are over-weight, there is a measure of personal or environmental influence.

Our modern culture is such that most of us cannot resist trying to tweak our weight a bit. Nearly half of Americans consider themselves overweight, and on any given day, roughly 40 percent of women and 23 percent of men are trying to lose weight—usually by dieting. But of course saying that weight is partially within our control is by no means the same as saying that losing weight or even preventing a gain is easy.

TWO

Of Mice and Men

THE DISCOVERY OF
AN OBESITY GENE

One day during the summer of 1949 an unusual creature arrived in the bustling seaside town of Bar
Harbor, Maine. At that time, Bar Harbor was used to
attracting extraordinary citizens. Millionaires, movie
stars, and international tourists had all been flocking to
this summering place for socialites for over a century. This
creature, however, belonged to a different class entirely. It
was a roly-poly baby mouse.

The weights of newborn mice have never been the
stuff of announcements the way human baby weights are,
so no one remembers exactly how heavy this mouse was
when it emerged from its mother's womb. But its burgeoning weight in the weeks that followed caught the
attention of the animal caretakers where it was born, at
the Jackson Laboratory, two miles south of downtown Bar
Harbor.

The Jackson Laboratory is an institution that was built around a strong and incredibly foresightful vision: mice, as mammals, could be used to study hereditary traits and diseases in people. The laboratory opened in 1929. This was long before the structure of DNA was discovered, before scientists knew how genes were passed from one generation to the next. But the lab's founder, Clarence Cook Little, knew that some diseases appeared more often in some families than others, and he believed that looking at strains of inbred mice was a way of understanding a host of human conditions.

Little cajoled patrons for the funding for a little laboratory by the sea in Maine where, in the days before air-conditioning, the summers were cool enough that animals could be bred year-round. The tight-knit band of researchers he assembled there pitched in to survive the hardships of the Depression, voluntarily cutting their salaries by two-thirds, growing their own food, and gradually turning a profit by selling to other labs the mice they bred from their purebred stocks. Eventually, when World War II broke out, one of the lab's biggest customers became the U.S. government, which bought thousands of mice a week for tests of the diseases that American troops were being exposed to in the Pacific theater.

In October of 1947 a great fire struck Bar Harbor. For ten days it raged through the coastal community, and after an unexpected shift of winds a wall of fire assaulted the lab. None of the scientists was hurt, as they had escaped by car and boat to safety. But the wooden mouse cages, beset by bedbugs since almost the opening of the lab, had routinely been treated with creosote and kerosene. As a result some 60,000 mice perished in an instant conflagration. Yet the importance of the Jackson Lab as a scientific resource had been established. The research community was used to getting their mouse stocks from the lab and now returned some of their colonies to restock Jackson.

By 1949, although the front steps of the lab had still not been replaced, the mouse production department was back in full swing. So many mice were being bred that mutations sprang up almost daily, and it was the special task of the research assistants who took care of the animals to spot interesting new traits. Ann Ingalls was one of the caretakers. At the time, she was working with George Snell, a geneticist who went on to win a Nobel Prize for his work on immunology. One day during the routine work of sorting through Snell's mouse stocks, Ingalls spotted a female animal that was a little plumper than normal. The mouse had extra-fuzzy fur—the result of a mutation that had already been seen. But there was something more.

Ingalls conferred with Margaret Dickie, a dark-haired woman with a crooked smile who was doing her doctoral research on mouse hormones. Together they decided that the mouse was probably just pregnant. They plucked it out of its cage and set it aside for further observation. Over the weeks that followed, they watched the mouse grow bigger and bigger until it was five times the size of its mouse cousins. By then they realized that this mouse wasn't pregnant at all. It was simply fat.

It ate three times the food of a normal mouse. Instead of a typical 10-minute burst of feeding, it would pound on the bar of the food hopper for two or three hours at a time. Later research showed that even if it was fed the same amount as a normal mouse, it still got fat. The only exercise it did was reaching up to the food hopper, and it had problems moving around because of its weight.

Clearly, its sedentary nature was a factor in its obesity. But during the periods of time when it wasn't eating it would go into a kind of torpor. Its body temperature dropped and so did its oxygen consumption. It seemed to be conserving energy very effectively, taking what looked like short bouts of hibernation. This was an animal destined to expand. And even amid the motley collection of mice at the Jackson Labs, such a trait was exceedingly rare.

There was only one other genetically fat mouse known to scientists at that time, an animal that its discoverers named *agouti* because its particular brand of obesity went hand in hand with a mottled yellow coat similar to the fur of the agouti rodents of South America and the West Indies. Both the *agouti* mouse and the newly discovered mouse at Jackson shared the distinction of having their excess weight boil down to a single gene—one scrap of DNA, whose sequence of base pairs coded for a crucial protein. If a mouse lacked this protein, the animal's entire weight-control machinery went awry, making it fat. In finding the heavy mouse, the Jackson scientists opened a new door on one of the enduring mysteries of biology—how animals, and by extension people, keep weight in check. Several months after the discovery, Dickie danced into the lab director's office waving a copy of the *Journal of Heredity* over her head. The plump mouse had made the cover of the December 1950 issue. Ingalls, Dickie, and Snell called this brand new genetic variation *obese*, a name that was later shortened to *ob* (pronounced "o.b.").

The *ob* mouse came into a world that was already quite concerned about excess weight. Although fat was nowhere near the obsession it is today, 1948 saw the launch of TOPS, or Take Off Pounds Sensibly, the first of many group dieting organizations to emerge across the United States in the postwar period. The founder of TOPS, Milwaukee housewife Esther Manz, read an article on Alcoholics Anonymous and became convinced that a mutually supportive environment would be just as beneficial to people struggling with their weight. With three friends gathered around her kitchen table, she convened the first TOPS session. In time, however, her program blossomed into a vast network of group meetings where those who lost weight were literally crowned as royalty and those who didn't were often just as grandly scorned.

This polarized view of weight drew strength from all corners of society, from the influential world of fashion to the medical profession. In the prosperous decade following the war, many women amassed not only the money but the time and the desire to follow fashion trends. They democratized what was once an upper-class world of French couturiers and the elite fashion press. Thus, when Christian Dior's New Look made its debut on Paris runways in 1947, it launched a fashion revolution that was felt on all rungs of the social ladder. Gone were the square shoulders and straight lines of the war years. Dior's full skirts and soft, sloping shoulders placed a renewed emphasis on the "feminine" shape. Yet that didn't mean that most women's shapes were suited to it. As Dior himself once said, the New Look required "handspan waists."

If the effort to squeeze themselves into fashionable garb wasn't enough to convince mid-century women to slim down, fat's bad medical reputation provided an additional argument. In 1952 the director of the National Institutes of Health declared obesity to be the nation's number one nutrition problem. And just like today, supposedly "scientific" cures promising to help people shed their unhealthy pounds were everywhere.

One of the most popular was a low-calorie liquid diet known as Metrecal. Metrecal was that era's version of the chocolatey Slimfast shakes pitched on TV today by everyone from former Los Angeles Dodgers manager Tommy Lasorda to small-screen celebrity Ann Jillian. Though the Mead Johnson Company didn't launch it onto the market until 1959, the shake was based on a formula that had already been part of the dieter's world for years.

The roots of this dubious diet food lay in scientific research conducted at New York's Rockefeller University during the early 1950s. Doctors there who were studying metabolism had experimented with a low-calorie mixture of ingredients that resembled the basic protein-carbohy-drate-fat ratios in breast milk. The research was picked up by two women's magazines, *Vogue* and *Ladies Home Journal*, leading to a do-it-yourself fad of mixing together dextrose, evaporated milk, oil, and water into an all-in-one diet drink.

As the historian Hillel Schwartz pointed out in his impressive cultural history of dieting, *Never Satisfied*, this fabulous formula not only satisfied the appetite but also addressed the deeper needs of the heart by returning consumers to the most satisfying of all experiences, suckling at their mother's breast. Such a solution to dieters' woes could hardly have been more appropriate to the era. Freud's theories on the nature of the unconscious had a firm grip on the 1950s psyche. Fat was variously seen as a way to shield oneself against the outside world or the result of subsuming the traits of an overbearing mother. Either choice left people with the conviction that the problem of overweight was primarily psychological. They were fat because unconscious motives were driving them to overeat.

Xavier Pi-Sunyer began his medical career when such ideas were in fashion. Now director of Columbia University's Obesity Research Center and editor of the journal *Obesity Research*, he is one of the most respected voices in the field. He brings to the table both the wisdom and the humility that four decades of experience with treating overweight patients have given him. I asked him during an interview in his office to look back on the scientific concepts that influenced obesity treatment at mid-century.

"The old tradition that obese people are psychiatrically ill turned out to be totally wrong," he said as the late afternoon sunlight streamed across his desk. "For years psychiatrists have been treating obese patients and psychoanalyzing them and saying that they have to get their act together emotionally before they will be able to solve their obesity problem. . . . In fact obese people time and time again have been shown to have no more psychiatric illness than anybody else. And if they're depressed, a lot of it is related to the way people treat them."

Pi-Sunyer admitted during our conversation that the link between eating and emotions was something he still hadn't worked out to his satisfaction. "Patients do tell you that when they're upset they eat more; that when they're elated they eat more; that there are a lot of mood swings that focus them on eating. But whether that's a reaction to an internal biological drive that they then interpret as emotion is not clear to me. We know that emotions are genetically determined. If your parents are depressed you have a much larger chance of being depressed yourself. So I'm not sure it's very helpful to talk about food intake as being emotional."

The fact that mid-century scientists talked about obesity in this way, however, was something he readily explained. "Traditionally, when medicine or biology doesn't know something, they say it's due to psychiatric problems or emotions." A number of conditions, from hemophilia to Gulf War syndrome, have gone through the same process.

Thus the 1950s public, having been sold the psychoanalytic view that with enough work, anything could be changed, logged thousands of hours in therapy. With this rush to the analyst's couch, the nature-nurture pendulum made a pronounced swing toward the latter. The old idea that obesity was a glandular disease—the result of such things as faulty thyroid organs—fell by the wayside. Similarly, genetic explanations for obesity were thought to apply in only a few rare cases.

That being the case, it is easier to understand why medical researchers of that era didn't seize on the newly discovered *ob* mouse as a tool to help them understand obesity. Weight gain was a psychological problem, not a physiological one. Instead, researchers saw potential in the *ob* mouse for understanding a more strictly medical condition: type II diabetes. They had known for some time that obesity often went hand in hand with this disease. If the portly mouse was going to be of any use to medicine, it would be as an animal model for the study of diabetes.

That was the thinking of nutritionist Jean Mayer, the late president of Tufts University, who heard about the *ob* mouse at a conference at Jackson soon after it was discovered. He ordered *ob* mice as fast as the animal caretakers could breed them and ship them to his lab, then at the Harvard School of Public Health. As he had hoped, the animals showed early promise. Mayer learned that they did indeed have the high blood sugar and insulin resistance characteristic of diabetes in people. But then as time went on he found that these traits gradually disappeared from the breeding stock, and his hope turned to frustration. "He would complain all the time how they couldn't get diabetic mice anymore," recalled Jackson biochemist Doug Coleman.

Coleman, who recently retired after a distinguished career at the lab, began working there in the late 1950s when demand for *ob* was languishing. "I was always kind of interested in the *obese* mouse," he said in a recent interview. "I thought it was kind of a pity that nobody was really looking at it because it seemed to have some interesting potential. But I was doing other things." At the time, Coleman was immersed in the study of mice with muscular dystrophy.

The turning point in his career came with a chance appearance of another fat mouse in the breeding stocks. This mouse looked and acted just like the earlier one. It even had diabetic traits. But pedigree searches and breeding tests quickly made it clear that the DNA mutation that caused the second mouse to gain weight was entirely different from the one in *ob*.

That was enough to hook Coleman. He set to work analyzing the new animal. Rather than just present the discovery as another fat mouse that also had diabetes, Coleman wanted to describe it as thoroughly as possible. He and his colleagues soon learned that what they actually had were two unique mice, *ob* and the new one, which Coleman dubbed *diabetic*, or *db*. Both types behaved the same way but for different reasons, a fact that Coleman made profoundly clear with an elegant if somewhat grisly set of experiments.

Coleman surgically joined the bloodstreams of pairs of mice using a procedure called parabiosis. The technique involves cutting down the bellies of the animals, through their coats, and then sewing the cuts together so that some of the capillaries meld. The trick was to suture the shoulders of the two animals together so that they didn't pull themselves apart, Coleman once told me over

Thai food, in the same matter-of-fact tone he used to order a salad. He was leaning on his elbows, delivering a rapid-fire soliloquy about the experiments with all the details of an immediate memory in spite of the fact that some two decades had passed.

When Coleman joined the animals in this way, they didn't exchange a lot of blood—only about 1 percent. But this was enough to have an effect. When *obese* mice were joined to normal mice, they stopped their eating sprees and their weights never ballooned. The reason seemed straightforward to Coleman. Something in the normal animal's bloodstream was telling it when to stop eating. The *obese* mice weren't producing this signal on their own, but they could recognize it when it drifted over from the blood of the normal animal.

In contrast, the *diabetic* mice manufactured plenty of this satiety signal, so much that when *db* mice were joined to normal mice, the normal mouse would shrink to the point of starvation. The same thing happened when *db* mice were joined to the *ob* mice. Again, Coleman saw the light. The problem with the *diabetic* mouse was that it simply wasn't getting the satiety message. It was flooding its bloodstream with the signal, but it could not recognize the compound, and it gained weight just like the *obese* mouse.

All of this Coleman had figured out by 1978. But in spite of putting in a great deal of additional work describing the *ob* and *db* mice, Coleman never got any closer to understanding just what was missing from the animals' bloodstreams that caused them to get fat. "I spent twenty years trying to track down this mysterious factor," he said wistfully, "but the technology just wasn't ready at that time."

The Seventies

While Coleman toiled, the 1970s saw many obesity researchers turning their attention toward a new type of treatment called behavioral therapy. Behaviorism was a new idea sweeping through the field of psychology. It threw out all the Freudian stuff about unconscious motives and focused instead on the tangible. What mattered to behaviorists were people's actions and their reactions to various situations.

Behaviorism had evolved out of the frustration that psychologists felt with their inability to say anything concrete about mental processes. Unable to see inside the human brain, they couldn't shed much light on how the gray matter gives rise to the myriad thoughts and feelings we all possess. But one thing researchers could observe were actions—physical responses to specific conditions inside the laboratory.

The Russian physiologist Ivan Pavlov had set the ball in motion with his groundbreaking work on dogs. He showed that he could condition them to drool spontaneously at the sound of a dinner bell. Such "conditioned reflexes" provided a new way of studying brain activity, and the work earned Pavlov a Nobel Prize in 1904.

Half a century later, the psychologist B. F. Skinner applied these ideas to people. He reasoned that if an animal's actions could be triggered reliably by a certain stimulus, then people might be similarly conditioned. He didn't really expect people to behave in exactly the same way every time he presented them with a stimulus. But he showed that with enough reinforcement, he could increase the probability that an event would trigger the desired reaction.

Then in the late 1960s, Richard Stuart at the University of Michigan's School of Social Work pressed the behaviorists' ideas into service to help people control their eating. Stuart took a handful of overweight patients and asked them to write down what they ate and drank as well as the time of day and the circumstances that surrounded each meal. He then looked through these diaries for the conditions that caused these people to overeat or eat unhealthily.

When patients ate in front of the television, for instance, he speculated that they might be less aware of how much they were eating and might consume a great deal by the time they realized they were full. In contrast, if they read during a meal they might eat less overall. When such connections became clear, Stuart encouraged people to reinforce the environments that gave them positive results.

"Behavior modification worked better than psychoanalysis," said Pi-Sunyer. "It was very concrete and very straightforward and you worked on, essentially, tasks." It quickly became the hot new treatment strategy for obesity researchers frustrated by psychotherapy's record of failure at helping people lose weight. By 1975, a hundred scientific papers and countless books on the subject of behavioral therapy had appeared. In the hands of thoughtful practitioners it was and still can be an effective method of helping people gradually acquire healthy habits of eating and exercise.

Over the years, however, the effectiveness of behavioral therapy has been unwittingly diluted by its practitioners. It has become most widely known for the second branch of Stuart's treatment method. In addition to keeping diaries, Stuart's subjects learned a handful of behaviors that were intended to help them reach the goal of eating less. Eat slowly. Put the fork down after each bite. Pause during a meal. Do all your eating in one place.

To veterans of the weight wars, these dictums may strike a familiar chord. The series of tricks to slow the act of eating became a mantra for many dieters. Perhaps because of their simplicity, they eventually eclipsed the other aspects of the treatment. At its most quick and dirty, behavioral therapy evolved into giving patients a handout listing the rules of eating and then leaving the rest up to them. Thus behavioral therapy may have taken away the Freudian emphasis on underlying desires. But in the end it often replaced them with an obsessive attention to eating habits.

Compounding that increased eating awareness was a burgeoning body consciousness in American society during the decade of the 1970s. Who can forget fluffy-haired Farrah Fawcett in the red bathing suit poster that went on to become one of the best selling pin-ups of all time? Farrah's swimsuit was scarcely more revealing than that of her predecessor, Betty Grable, but her figure was substantially slimmer, an impossible target for most women to meet.

Saturday Night Fever swept the nation's cinemas in the late 1970s, giving a boost to clingy disco leotards. It took good bodies to wear these freer, slinkier fashions, and for women in particular those bodies had to stand on their own merits. This was the era of bra burning, after all— though many will be surprised to learn that girdles were the undergarments women scorned most. Sales of girdles, and to a lesser extent brassieres, plummeted throughout the decade.

Without the crutch foundation garments provided, many women—as well as men—took up jogging to keep in shape. James Fixx's *The Complete Book of Running* became an instant bestseller when it appeared in 1977. The hardcover edition alone sold a million copies. The same year, 47 percent of Americans claimed to be exercising regularly, more than double the number in the early 1960s. "Body nazis" and "runner's high" began to pepper our vocabulary.

Biology Comes of Age

The 1970s were also a historic decade for molecular biology. During a scientific meeting in 1973, Herbert Boyer, a biologist at the University of California in San Francisco, revealed to his colleagues that he and Stanley Cohen at Stanford had developed a technique for putting foreign genes into bacteria. With that successful exchange, genetic engineering was born. Before long, genes from almost any organism could be spliced into the DNA of any other organism, from bacteria to mice to men. By a process similar to the production of beer, substances like human insulin were soon being manufactured for the treatment of diabetics.

Throughout the decade, biologists were also using the techniques of genetic engineering—of breaking the DNA open at specific spots and then sticking the loose ends together again—to explore the human genome the way a toddler tests a plastic chain of links. While they were tinkering, they discovered that a series of unique markers lies sprinkled throughout the vast expanse of human DNA. The markers are short DNA sequences that repeat themselves. The sequences can repeat a couple of times in one person and several dozen times in another person. With the discovery of these repeats, biologists suddenly had a fantastic new tool for finding genes.

Prior to that, trying to locate an unknown gene was like looking for a specific billboard along the 3,000-mile stretch of highway between New York and San Francisco by walking from one end to the other and simply keeping your eyes peeled. In other words, biologists might find what they were looking for by testing every gene along the entire length of a chromosome, but the search would take an incredibly long time. The genetic markers offered an alternative. Researchers could use them to first narrow down the search to a reasonably small stretch of DNA and then explore the stretch in more detail. Markers made finding genes practical. Biologists quickly seized on these markers to probe the genetic roots of all manner of human traits and afflictions.

Jeffrey Friedman was one such biologist. Tall, with a halo of curly brown hair, he grew up on Long Island and graduated from medical school at the tender age of 22. By 1986, he was starting his own research laboratory at Rockefeller University and looking around for a fresh, absorbing project to launch his career. He had long been interested in the topic of behavior. As a biologist, he thought of behavior not as some mysterious, evanescent quality, but largely as a product of our biochemistry and our genes. He saw that the dramatic advances of the last decade had finally given researchers the tools to answer deeper questions about why people act they way they do.

In particular Friedman wanted to look at eating behavior. Eating is clearly a complex phenomenon influenced not only by the physical need to fuel the body but also by a person's environment, mood, and upbringing, among many other factors. In that way it is similar to many of the human animal's most intriguing and mysterious behaviors, from the tendency toward violence to a susceptibility to mental illnesses like depression and schizophrenia. Unlike these other aspects of personality, however, the act of eating can present a fairly straightforward quantity to measure not only in people but in laboratory animals.

During Friedman's early training as a scientist he had done some research on a compound in our bodies called cholecystokinin that influences how much food we eat. At the time he had thought it might be the key to what was going wrong with the *ob* mouse's weight-control system. That turned out not to be the case. But the idea of using eating to look at the biological basis of behavior in general was still stuck in his mind when he went to a seminar in the mid-1980s in which Lou Kunkel, a molecular geneticist at Children's Hospital in Boston, talked about his search for the gene for muscular dystrophy.

"It was pretty clear from that that they were going to be able to identify the MD gene," said Friedman during an interview in 1995. "And it just seemed to me that if you could clone a mutant gene out of the human, if anything, it ought to be easier in a mouse. So it raised the possibility that similar methods could be used to find *ob*."

Back at the lab he put together a plan for finding the gene that made the *ob* mouse fat. Friedman's plan wasn't terribly different from the techniques used to identify the genes for muscular dystrophy, cystic fibrosis, and what is now a rapidly increasing list of human diseases. It had been known for some time that the *ob* gene was on mouse chromosome 6. Friedman was going to narrow down the location of the gene to a specific region of the chromosome, fish out the genes in that region, and test them to see whether they were the ones that were mutated in the *ob* animals.

On paper, the plan was straightforward, but it concealed a wealth of difficulties. The first hurdle Friedman encountered was the fact that not that many genes had been mapped in mice. As a result, the infrastructure for doing such work wasn't nearly as well developed as it was for humans. A lot of the early research in his laboratory amounted to gruntwork that generated DNA markers that simply did not exist for mice, although human versions had been in use for years.

This work narrowed the location of the gene down to a segment of DNA between two markers, Pax 4 and D6 Rck 13. Friedman's team didn't know the exact length of the segment, but the markers provided good starting points for their search. The next step was to walk along the DNA between these two markers until they found the exact gene.

In fact, a "chromosome walk," as the technique is now commonly called, is more like trying to lay down train track while simultaneously riding on it. To make the pieces of the track, Friedman's team cut up the DNA between the two markers into many shorter segments. These pieces overlapped each other, but unlike standard train track they would fit together only in a predetermined order.

To begin their walk, the researchers used the sequences of the two markers to pick out pieces of DNA track that contained matching sequences. From there, they had to find pieces whose ends overlapped the pieces they had already laid. That meant finding the sequences at the ends of the two known pieces and then using the ends to fish out new pieces. In this way the researchers carried out dozens of time-consuming steps, laying one piece of track after another after another until, finally, they had covered the entire region of DNA between Pax 4 and D6 Rck 13.

Each time they sequenced the ends of one of these DNA pieces, they also used the piece to see how close they were getting to the *ob* gene. In doing so, they took advantage of an unusual property of genes. Scientists have known for some time that even though the position of a gene along a chromosome doesn't change, what lies next to it can vary from one generation to the next. This isn't some biological riddle, but merely a result of the genetic mixing that goes on when egg and sperm cells are formed.

Although everyone has two copies of a gene—one from each parent—only one of the copies is passed on to the next generation. Which one depends on a mysterious dance in which parallel chains of DNA seem to crisscross and swap some of their genetic material. Genes that are side by side tend to travel together during these swaps. The farther apart two genes are, the more likely they are to be separated. Biologists can exploit this process to figure out whether a certain marker is close to a gene. Markers that travel with the gene from one generation to the next are presumed to be nearer—they are "linked."

Thus, Friedman and his team would look at the offspring from hundreds of mouse matings to see whether the end sequence had traveled with the *ob* gene. When they found linkage, they knew they were getting closer to *ob*. In this way they narrowed down the segment containing the obese gene to a critical region of 650,000 letters on the DNA chain. From this region, they then began to tease out individual genes.

Which of these was the *ob* gene? To limit the possibilities, the researchers began to look at where the product of each gene, the RNA, was being made inside the mouse's body. If the RNA was only in the lungs or the heart or any of the other organs not directly involved in metabolism or food storage, then the researchers figured the chances were good that the gene wasn't *ob* and they could set it aside. Anything else was a potential candidate.

One day, RNA for one of the genes they were testing showed up only in fat. "I must say that fat was not my first choice as a likely organ," Friedman confessed to an audience at Harvard Medical School in 1996 as he told them the story of the discovery. "I always thought the liver would be a likely sight of synthesis for a molecule regulating nutritional state. But of course, we didn't ignore the possibility that this gene was indeed a good candidate. And so with this knowledge in hand . . . we quickly did the next experiment."

The researchers looked for RNA from this gene in *ob* mice. The result couldn't have been clearer. The animals' fat tissue wasn't producing any RNA from the gene at all. The missing compound had to be what was causing the mice to be fat. At this point Friedman knew in his heart that the gene was indeed *ob*. But definitive proof lay in sequencing the gene in both the normal and the *ob* animals to show a gene defect in the *obese* mice. Months passed as the researchers amassed the evidence that they had located the *ob* gene.

In May 1994, eight years after forging his original plan, Friedman went out to dinner with Doug Coleman and a Rockefeller colleague, Rudy Leibel, who was working on a related mouse project. Such get-togethers were routine when Coleman came to New York for a meeting. But that night, Coleman remembers, "Jeff was walking visibly a foot off the ground. So I said, 'Jeff, you know you're not telling me something. You told me always that I'd be the first to know.' And he said, 'Well I've just done the *obese* gene.' And he said, 'Everything you predicted was absolutely right.'"

Friedman's paper about the mouse appeared in the December 1, 1994 issue of the scientific journal *Nature*. It located the *ob* gene and showed that it failed to produce a functioning protein in *ob* mice. Friedman later dubbed the protein leptin from the Greek *leptos*, meaning thin. News of the discovery appeared in newspapers throughout the country the same day alongside pictures of the *ob* mouse on a scale, outweighing two of its lean cousins. Memorable though this image was, what made the discovery front-page news was not so much the gene's presence in mice but the fact that the researchers had found a strikingly similar gene in people.

All at once, skinny became not a moral high ground but a genetic legacy. This news resonated for a public that had already witnessed a multitude of gene discoveries. Traits like anxiety, introversion, drug addiction, and sexual preference have all been pinned on genes in recent years. A belief that genes control human behavior and ability has swept our late twentieth-century culture.

This swing of the nature-nurture pendulum, like all those of the past, is undoubtedly a passing phase. Neither inheritance nor upbringing can be dismissed from the array of influences that make us human. As the evolutionary biologist Stephen J. Gould pointed out in a recent essay, the only meaningful way to talk about nature and nurture these days is in terms of their interactions: how the environment of the womb, for example, affects gene development; how genes predispose us to greet different learning environments. But when it comes to weight, questions of nature versus nurture are more than intellectual exercises. Anything that sheds light on why and what we weigh and what we can do about it is the stuff of daily life.

The *ob* discovery not only introduced to millions of people the idea that fat could be inherited, it also raised the possibility that people could be given leptin to help them lose weight. Friedman knew from Coleman's experiments that the protein this gene produced somehow let an animal's body know that it had eaten enough. His theory was that it did so, in both mice and people, by telling the brain how much fat was in the body's stores. The early thinking was that people who were obese might be given this protein if their bodies were not making enough. However, further research soon toppled the idea that a lack of leptin was a common problem.

In an informal test during the weeks following the gene discovery, Friedman looked at leptin levels in blood samples from half a dozen members of his laboratory, including himself. Friedman is a relatively lean man. At that time he showed the highest circulating levels of leptin ever recorded. Yet no one has been able to explain the result, other than to chalk it up to poetic justice. For as researchers in the coming months measured leptin levels in more than six people, it became clear that, in general, the more fat people have on their bodies the higher their blood levels of leptin.

In fact, most obese people had too much leptin floating around their bodies. Their excess weight seemed to stem from their resistance to this signal. Whether giving them a drug that would boost leptin levels even further would have any effect on their weight remained to be seen. But in all likelihood, an effective drug would have to help people overcome the resistance, and that would require a good deal more developmental research. These were only some of the hurdles encountered by scientists who saw the leptin discovery as the beginning of a new era for antiobesity medications. The *ob* breakthrough touched on many charged issues of how our culture deals with fat—not the least of which was whether obese people *need* to take drugs to change the way they look.

That issue came up often during the media scramble to analyze the *ob* gene discovery. On the day the *Nature* paper came out, Friedman appeared live on television's CNN. The other guest on the program was Frances White, president of the National Association to Advance Fat Acceptance, a group that works to eradicate the stigma attached to being obese. White's position on the discovery was that it proved something that fat people had long maintained—body weight is merely a trait, like height, that characterizes each of us. The problem, said White, was that society stigmatizes people on the basis of appearance.

CNN's interviewer, Reid Collins, challenged White. "It is agreed generally, isn't it, that overweight is a danger to one's health?" "Now would you say that no thin person has high blood pressure?" White responded. "No thin person is prone to heart disease? I don't think so. So of course my concern about this is, is this going to be some magic pill that is supposed to be crammed down my throat so that I can conform to a societal pressure to change my looks, when that societal standard changes every generation?"

She had raised one of the key issues in the ongoing effort to treat obesity medically. And in fact, Friedman took her side, saying that whether or not obesity requires treatment is a health issue, not an aesthetic one. Yet aesthetics, White pointed out, are what the issue of fat discrimination is all about.

"But the doctors helped you now," the interviewer offered. "You can say, 'It's in my genes, I'm not responsible.'" Indeed that was the trump card many people saw in the *ob* gene discovery. It lent support to the argument that fat people are born, not made. It shot holes in the stereotypical view of the obese as lazy gluttons.

Yet even the interviewer's statement appeared to White to be loaded with cultural bias. Collins had implied that excess weight was something for which White needed an excuse, and she wasn't having any of it. Scientists have isolated genes that contribute to tallness, she pointed out. "And quite frankly, tall people don't live as long as people of average height. But I don't notice anybody saying that Michael Jordan has a genetic defect . . . the way you are describing me now."

Such issues of whether obesity is truly a health threat and whose business it is to worry about weight anyway have continued to rage in the years since the *ob* gene discovery. At the same time, *ob* has opened the gate to a flood of new research on obesity. The leptin protein is turning out to be a key component in the body's weight control system—more central than researchers dared hope when the compound was first described.

The notoriety that has surrounded each new leptin finding has only added to Friedman's prestige. If the Mafia concept of a "made man" can be applied to science, Friedman is now one of them. Yet fame in science is still a relative phenomenon. At a gathering of his fellow biologists three months after the *ob* gene discovery, Friedman opened his talk with a story that brought his 15 minutes into focus.

"When our paper came out," he said, "it received a lot of attention from the lay press. And I was sort of nervous about the whole thing and was trying to keep at a distance. But I must confess that one day it occurred to me that perhaps someone on the street whom I didn't know would recognize me. And so I admit that was a little vain, but I was walking around the streets of New York making eye contact with a lot of people, which is quite dangerous." Friedman paused to let the audience appreciate the image.

"Nothing happened the first day and the second day. Then on the third day I was walking—I had just finished playing tennis with [Rockefeller biologist] Jim Darnell . . . and I'd just about given up. And as we were walking back to the university we passed a homeless guy on the street. He's lying on a piece of cardboard, and as I walk by he goes, 'Hey, you!'" Friedman imitated the gravelly voice. "So I ignore him. He says, 'Hey, you!' and I ignore him.

And five times he goes, 'Hey, you!' After the fifth time I turn around and I look at him and he goes, 'You're the asshole that was on TV last night!' He was the only person who recognized me. I don't think he thought I was on *Seinfeld* either."

THREE

No, They Can't Take That Away from Me

DIETING VERSUS NATURE

On a bright Saturday morning in November, at a television studio in Nashville, Gwen Shamblin sits atop a platform stage in a cozy, high-backed chair. She is tugging at the blonde tresses that rise above her forehead, repeatedly pulling the stack of hair higher and then smoothing it down. Her look of intense concentration looms large in the video monitors on either side of her, holding the attention of the crowd that fills the Tennessee studio's seats and aisles.

Shamblin is here to tape the fourth in a new series of videos for her Christian-based diet program, the Weigh Down Workshop. She covers her face while an assistant on stage douses her head with a cloud of aerosol spray. Then she begins to explain to her audience that she's trying to get her hair to look the way it did at the end of a segment taped earlier in the week.

"We've just had a cafe scene where we had a binge that was hilarious," she says, somehow knowing that out-of-control eating will strike this audience as funny. "The husband comes home, the wife throws the table cloth over the food and then dumps her laundry on top of it and starts to fold the laundry." Over the laughter she adds, "The cafe was called the Golden Cafe."

An appreciative murmur runs through the studio as audience members get the reference to the golden calf—the false God the Bible warns against worshipping. Both the folksy wordplay and the reference itself sum up Shamblin's philosophy of weight control. She believes that food is a false God. For her the problem of excess weight boils down to one key issue: People are overweight because they have a love affair with food.

"You dress for it. You put on your stretch clothes to make sure that nothing hinders you from that rendezvous with the refrigerator at ten o'clock at night," Shamblin told a rapt audience at Desert Oasis '97, the second national seminar for her diet program. "Until we admit that we are in love heart, soul, mind, and strength with food, we can never lose the weight permanently."

Shamblin's solution to this problem is for people to convert their love of food into love for God. "Transfer [the] urge for a pan of brownies to that of hungering and thirsting after righteousness," she says. In dispensing such self-help homilies, Shamblin is part of a growing trend.

Since the 1950s, Christian-based diets have made up an ever-increasing share of the diet-advice industry—a market of books, programs, foods and other weight-related products that nets over $34 billion a year in the United States alone. Fasting and deprivation have, of course, been part of the religious tradition for centuries. The Cornell University historian Joan Jacobs Brumberg has detailed the lives of many abstemious saints, from Catherine of Siena, who ate only herbs, to Eva Fleigen, the "Fasting Woman of Meurs." But the first book to openly preach the gospel of slimming was *Pray Your Weight Away* (1957), by Presbyterian minister Charlie Shedd.

That book paved the way for a boom in religious diet literature in the 1970s, with titles like *Help Lord—The Devil Wants Me Fat!* and Shedd's best-selling 1972 effort, *The Fat Is in Your Head*. These accompanied the rise of religious weight-watcher groups like Overeaters Victorious and 3D (for Diet, Discipline, and Discipleship), a program that was being offered in more than 5,000 churches around the country by 1981.

In today's multimedia era, religious diet advice is as popular as ever. Sheri Chambers's 1996 video "Praise Aerobics" has sold over 50,000 copies. First Place and Jesus is the Weigh are among the many Christian-based diet programs that have emerged and gone national during the 1980s and 1990s. Shamblin's Weigh Down Workshop, a 12-week Bible study program now offered in some 10,000 churches both in the United States and abroad, is currently the largest of these programs.

Like all diets with a religious focus, the Weigh Down Workshop has much the same allure as secular programs— the promise of freedom from unwanted pounds. It also taps into the inherent authority and epic sweep of Biblical narrative. Shamblin routinely compares the journey of Moses out of Egypt to the journey from the slavery of diets through the Desert of Testing. At the edge of this desert, across the River Jordan, is the Promised Land of no desire to overeat. God programmed us to know when we are hungry and when we are full, Shamblin teaches. If we can learn to heed these signals, He will deliver us from our excess weight.

Shamblin claims that her program can get anybody to the point where they can stop eating in the middle of a candy bar and never for a moment feel deprived. This is an intriguing proposition and one she repeats often in her promotional materials, partly for its sheer sales appeal and partly because within this promise lies the story of her own personal journey from weight-plagued coed to weight-loss guru.

A so-called "normal" eater as a girl, Shamblin says she began to get into trouble when she entered college. Both her love of food and the end of years of cheerleader practices added 20 pounds to her petite frame. Along the way, her intense focus on food led her to major in dietetics and nutrition. But she found the courses lacking because they failed to provide an explanation for why her grandparents could eat bacon and eggs every day as well as rich desserts like coconut cake and pecan pie and still maintain their ideal weights while she was looking more and more like "a potato with toothpick legs." Her studies were also lacking, she felt, because they made no mention of the Creator.

What she found much more enlightening during her college years were the results of a personal quest to figure out what was in the mind of a skinny friend that allowed her to eat only half a McDonald's quarter-pounder and then quit. Shamblin followed the girl around for a couple of days and never really found the answer. When asked why she hadn't finished a meal, the friend simply said she didn't want any more.

Shamblin decided to just imitate this "skinny" behavior, eating everything she was hungry for, but only when she was hungry. She soon dropped the excess pounds she had gained, and in the years that followed, skinny eating became a trusted friend to her whenever she ran into weight problems. It helped her lose the 50 pounds she gained while she was carrying her first child as well as the weight she put on with the subsequent pregnancies.

In the midst of the childbearing years Shamblin also began to combine her training in dietetics and her Christian faith to conduct a series of weight-loss classes for her local church. She saw many people lose weight, but then, as with most diet programs, they gained the weight back. These early failures focused her thinking. Still not knowing why she was able to stop eating mid-meal, only that she was, she looked to God for the answer. And the result of those prayers is the weight-loss program that has gained in popularity ever since, aided by her 1997 book, *The Weigh Down Diet*.

So many people want a higher authority to tell them what they should eat in order to lose weight that the idea of a diet sanctified by a religion can strike them as a literal godsend. At the same time, intellectuals can easily dismiss programs like Shamblin's as so much mumbo jumbo.

Somewhere between these two extremes lies the truth about the Weigh Down Diet.

Even more than most secular diet programs, it speaks to our nagging belief that our struggle with weight reflects a deep-seated unhappiness and lack of fulfillment. Shamblin sees the problem of overeating as primarily psychological—feeding head hunger instead of stomach hunger. She concludes that the way for someone to combat excess weight is to seek out what they are craving emotionally.

Among obesity researchers, just how large a role psychological and spiritual well-being play in our weight is still hotly debated. Yet most of them agree that the problems of overeating out of boredom or turning to food when we are anxious are undeniably real. And for those who believe, Shamblin's return to the Christian faith can truly be a source of solace.

An extraordinary sense of peace emanated from the dieters who offered weight-loss testimonials for Shamblin's Tennessee taping. Many other diet programs offer such testimonials from the formerly fat. Yet often people burst into tears the minute they get in front of an audience, as all the pain of their struggle wells up from just beneath the surface. Or their voices buzz with grim determination, as if their clenched teeth are the only thing that stands in the way of a relapse. The successful dieters on Shamblin's stage were calm and centered. Although there is no question that they were specially selected for this taping, they seemed more genuine in many ways than Shamblin herself.

Besides shining a light on the spiritual side of overeating, the Weigh Down program also forces a hard look at what is scientific fact and what is merely wishful thinking in any diet, Christian or otherwise. The vast majority of weight-loss schemes attempt to overrule or fool the body's weight-control mechanism—a challenging and invariably frustrating battle. Now more than ever, obesity researchers grasp the enormous power of our defense against deprivation. To Shamblin's credit, her religious program is one of the few to fall in line with this scientific understanding. Rather than fight the body with a restriction diet, it harnesses the hunger and satiety signals that lie dormant within us.

"Diets do not work because they are basically just making the food behave," writes Shamblin, "When we have taken out the sugar and replaced it with an artificial sugar, thrown out the fat and replaced it with an artificial fat, thrown out the calories and replaced them with noncaloric fluff or indigestible hay, we have made the food behave or change. We have not changed our own behavior. . . . Weigh Down is different from other programs because it is not selling a diet plan, a food, or whatever. It is a learning process. First, you understand hunger. Second, you recognize fullness and begin to stop at that point. Third, you develop the ability to sense what your body is really calling for."

Such commonsense rules of eating are a breath of fresh air in a world of carbohydrate exchanges and diet diaries. At the same time, one can hardly ignore the more troubling aspects of the Weigh Down Diet. Good old-fashioned evangelical guilt, when applied to eating, is enough to make many people, regardless of their faith, deeply suspicious. One of the most obvious problems with equating dieting and devotion to God in the lives of everyday sinners is that when people fail to lose weight, they see their weakness as more than just an insult to themselves. Not only do they regret their lack of will power, they also feel that they have transgressed the word of God. To Shamblin, this double whammy of shame is the strength of her program. She often tells her devotees that guilt is the punishment God has programmed into us to make us behave and do as He wishes. While few would question that this is her heartfelt belief, it is suspect at best and, at worst, unthinkably cruel.

Furthermore, while Shamblin may have her mind on heaven, she has her eyes on the bottom line. She made this patently clear in the first incarnation of the Weigh Down Workshop's online newsletter, which made a point of explaining to readers just how *The New York Times* and *Publishers' Weekly* create their best seller lists by surveying specific bookstores, "with the majority of their numbers coming from B. Dalton Booksellers and Waldenbooks." The newsletter suggested that the best way to glorify God would be to make the book a best-seller.

Such has been the fate of many diet books in recent years. *The New York Times*'s best-seller list has recently hosted *Dr. Atkins' New Diet Revolution*—a book, more than one obesity researcher has pointed out, that wouldn't have to have been written at all if his first book, *Dr. Atkins' Diet Revolution* (which sold over 10 million copies in the early 1970s), had worked. *Enter The Zone* by Barry Sears, which prescribes a similar high-protein regimen, has also been a smash hit with the diet book-buying public.

With all such weight-loss programs, their true worth lies in their long-term success—not on the best-seller list but in peoples' lives. For there are thousands of testimonials floating around by people who have lost massive amounts of weight. Nearly every dieter has some experience of a successful bout with weight. And the truth is that through sheer force of will, anyone can lose a substantial amount of weight.

Often diets help in the extraordinary effort of this task by limiting people to a few carefully selected foods. One popular regime that recently made the rounds of the dieters' samizdat network is the cabbage soup diet. It brought to mind the subtraction stew that was served in *The Phantom Tollbooth*. The more you ate, the hungrier you got. Cabbage and celery, which make up the bulk of the soup, are among those fabulous foods celebrated by dieters everywhere for taking as many calories to digest as they contain. The diet centered on eating unlimited quantities of this brew.

Other diets, rather than relying on one main food, keep people busy with the details of eating. Dieters are distracted with lists of acceptable foods, measurements of exact proportions, and specific combinations in which the foods can be eaten. A friend from Holland recently told me about her encounter with one such diet. She learned of it when many of the people at a dinner party she gave refused some of the dishes she served. My friend is a journalist, and she set out to investigate this new diet, which involved a lot of food pairing—foods that could be eaten only with certain other foods at particular times of the day. She sent the diet's prescribed rules of eating to a nutritionist and asked him whether this was indeed a good weight-loss program.

The nutritionist surprised her with his response. He said that he could give her a diet that allowed only foods that were, say, red and square and she would lose weight, not because the foods are inherently more nutritious or low in calories but because the diet forces her to jump through hoops. The attention required to select only foods that are red and then prepare them in a square form is a kind of barrier to the act of eating that can, in fact, help people lose weight. The food-pairing diet is similar, the nutritionist said. In short, fad diets achieve some measure of success because they cause people to limit their consumption of junk food as well as their intake of food in general.

High-protein diets like The Zone operate on a similar principle. This diet tells people to cut way down on carbohydrates and boost their intake of meat so that they get approximately 30 percent of their calories from protein and 40 percent from carbohydrates. For comparison, nutrition experts generally recommend getting 55 to 65 percent of calories from carbohydrates and 10 to 15 percent from protein. The rationale for this dietary change, according to the book's author, Barry Sears, is that carbohydrates cause an increase in insulin, and excess insulin causes the body to accumulate fat. The idea behind his diet is to keep insulin levels within a specific zone, causing the body to get rid of fat.

Eating carbohydrates does trigger the release of the hormone insulin into the bloodstream. The carbohydrates are broken down into a sugar called glucose. The insulin is a signal to brain and muscle cells to absorb this blood sugar, which then is either used as fuel or turned into fat. But obesity researchers say that Sears is wrong when he says that excess insulin makes you fat. Instead, the converse is true. Being fat causes many people to make excess insulin.

As we gain weight, our bodies pack more fat into our cells. As the cells fill up, they change shape and begin to shun the insulin signal to absorb more fuel. The bodies of many overweight people become "insulin resistant" and their blood sugar levels can become abnormally high. One-fourth of all Americans are insulin resistant. Most of these people won't lose weight by lowering their insulin levels but will lower their insulin levels by losing weight.

Insulin aside, what accounts for the fact that so many people are losing weight on the high-protein, low-carbohydrate diet? Obesity experts say that if people are losing on this diet, it is because they are cutting down on the total number of calories they consume. Chris Rosenbloom, a nutritionist at Georgia State University in Atlanta, has calculated that those who adhere to The Zone's rules are in fact on a low-calorie diet. Men are eating about 1,700 calories a day, women 1,300.

A low-calorie diet can lead to significant weight loss, regardless of what foods it labels as good and bad. But if there is one thing that health experts have learned in the last 50 years, it is that loading up on animal fat and protein is a recipe for health risks down the road. High-protein diets can spike cholesterol levels. In a study in which a small group of women followed Atkins's 1972 diet for two months, their levels of LDL (the bad cholesterol) rose by 33 percent, while their levels of HDL (the good kind) dropped 10 percent. Grains, beans, fruits, and vegetables are the best weapons we have to prevent heart disease and cancer. The limitations high-protein diets put on such essentially healthy foods are one of the major reasons why this and other high-protein diets don't make sense as long-term eating plans.

In addition, many high-protein diets are ketogenic—which means that they give the body so few carbohydrates to burn that it starts to burn fat. This would seem to be a cause for cheering. Yet the by-products of this process are chemicals called ketones, which the body works hard to flush out of its system.

Sears criticizes ketogenic diets in *Enter The Zone*, but Atkins celebrates ketosis. He calls it "one of life's charmed gifts." Since carbohydrates tend to store water in our bodies, the lack of them gives high-protein dieters an early and encouraging weight loss. The downside is that when our bodies excrete ketones they take sodium and potassium with them. Sodium loss can cause dehydration. Potassium loss can lead to cardiac arrhythmia. High-protein diets often result in weakness, nausea, and lightheadedness. Our bodies simply can't endure this peculiar regimen on a continuing basis. And as soon as people come off a high-protein diet and eat the carbohydrates their bodies crave, they quickly gain back the weight and the water they lost.

In the end, high-protein diets possess the same essential flaw common to most diets. What is in question is not whether they help us take weight off, but whether they train us to keep it off. Although our minds can override the biological urge to eat or to enjoy certain foods for a while, once our dedication to a diet wanes and our body's weight-regulating mechanisms become too strong to resist, we usually gain back the weight we lost—sometimes even a little extra.

As hard as it is to lose weight, keeping it off is even harder. Our bodies have evolved numerous ways to prevent us from growing leaner. These mechanisms are resistant to the sorts of tricks that dieters use to fool themselves into thinking they are eating more than they are. In fact, the more you know about the body's weight-control apparatus, the less likely you are to want to go on a diet.

Our Bodies Are Smarter Than We Think

In 1995 three scientists from Rockefeller University in New York published a study that showed how resistant our bodies are to weight loss. The idea that the body has a set weight that it defends—a set-point in the lingo of the obesity field—had been around since the 1950s. A host of studies since then have looked at what happened to the metabolisms of people who lost or gained weight, but their results disagreed. Some researchers found that dieters' bodies appeared to be counteracting a weight loss by conserving energy. Others found no change or even an increase in the amount of energy used. Likewise, no one knew what happened once people stabilized at a new, lower weight.

Rudolph Leibel, Michael Rosenbaum, and Jules Hirsch designed a study to answer these questions unequivocally. They recruited people who were obese as well as those who had never been overweight and studied them at an initial, stabilized weight as well as after they had changed weight. Some subjects lost 10 percent of their weight by consuming 800-calorie-a-day formula diets. Others gained 10 percent of their initial body weight by eating 5,000–8,000 calories a day. Whichever road they took, they stabilized their weights at the new plateau. Then the gainers dropped back down to their initial weights, stabilized, lost 10 percent, stabilized, and some of them even went on to lose 20 percent.

Throughout all these weight shifts, the researchers took careful measurements of how much energy the subjects expended. And indeed, the researchers found that when we lose pounds, our total energy use drops. It stays down for as long as our weights are reduced. Participants in the study who held their weight at 10 percent below their initial level showed a 15 percent drop in daily energy expenditure. Although the study did not specifically look at how long the drop in metabolism persisted, the researchers cited an earlier study by Leibel that showed that people who maintained a weight loss for periods of more than four years still showed reduced levels of energy expenditure.

The body is a remarkably efficient machine. When it takes in less fuel, it slows down. When it takes in more, it speeds up. This system helps keep body weight stable. When a person successfully loses weight and keeps it off, the body undergoes a change in metabolic rate. If too little fuel enters the system, the energy expenditure drops. If fuel intake increases, the body's metabolism quickens. The body modifies energy use so that weight is mostly steady. This works with people of naturally healthy weights or truly successful dieters.

One way the researchers suggested that the body might accomplish this stability is by changing how efficiently our muscles perform mechanical work. They found that weight loss had the largest effect on nonresting energy expenditure, which means the energy used during activities like walking and running that rely heavily on our muscles. If, as the researchers suggested, muscles become more efficient after a weight loss, then you have to work them more to expend the same amount of energy as before the weight drop. That may explain why exercise is helpful in maintaining a reduced body weight.

The other thing of particular interest about this study was that the researchers found this shift in metabolism to be just as marked after a weight gain as after a weight loss. Subjects who increased their weight showed 10 to 15 percent increases in their metabolism. Their bodies cranked up their energy use in order to help them take the excess pounds off.

To the average person struggling with weight, the latter finding sounds like poppycock. If our bodies are so good at adjusting metabolism for changes in weight, why do people get fat at all? What happened to the set-points of all of us who are carrying around an extra 20 pounds? These questions were addressed in an editorial that accompanied the publication of the study. William Ira Bennett, a physician at Cambridge Hospital in Cambridge, Massachusetts, wrote that the fact that we gain weight isn't proof that our bodies aren't defending a set-point. Rather, he said, the set-point can be reset by external factors. Things like our habitual levels of physical activity as well as the composition of our diets and how tasty or bland they are play a role in determining set-point.

In essence, the same sorts of diets that were mentioned in the first chapter as the ones that plump up the diet-induced obese mice can apply a gentle, upward pressure on our bodies' set-points. People may be eating only as much food as their bodies tell them they need. But Bennett's thesis is that the mere availability of rich, highly palatable food on a continuing basis can slowly increase the weight that the body is geared to defend. Some of us, he says, are especially susceptible to such pressure; others are resistant. Just which group we fall into, once again, boils down to our genes.

The fact is that until the nineteenth century, having too much food was never much of a health problem, which means that we evolved to be fairly lax about guarding against increases in the set-point. For obvious reasons, our bodies couldn't be so cavalier about decreases. A drop in weight had to be met with a full-court press lest the drop continue and lead eventually to death by starvation.

As a result, our bodies have developed a variety of defenses against going hungry. Shifts in metabolism like those the Rockefeller scientists measured are just one example. In fact, since the discovery of leptin, researchers are beginning to get a picture of the massive reorganization that takes place in many parts of the body when weight loss threatens. Like a nation faced with a siege, the starved body shuts down systems to conserve energy and simultaneously broadcasts the urgent need for more supplies.

Leptin is at the hub of many of these changes. This handy molecule does much more than just tell a mouse when it has eaten enough. While many researchers initially called leptin a "satiety signal" because of its role in the mouse, they quickly realized that leptin is also intimately involved in the body's defense against eating too little. In the broad scheme of things, shielding against starvation is much more useful to survival and is probably what the leptin molecule evolved to do.

Falling levels of leptin, says Jeff Flier, an endocrinologist at Beth Israel Hospital in Boston, send a signal that the body is getting too thin. Flier has shown that the body's reaction to this signal is widespread. The ovaries or testes of an animal that is put on a fast decrease their production of sex hormones, damping the animal's sex drive. Starving animals also turn down production of the thyroid hormones that tell their cells to burn food as fuel. Starvation boosts the production of stress hormones like cortisol, which helps an animal adapt to extreme deprivation by regulating bodily functions like blood pressure.

Replacing leptin prevents all these starvation-related activities.

Leptin levels also appear to be linked to a delay in the onset of puberty that comes as a result of starvation in animals and low body fat in people. A study of girls aged 8 to 13, which recorded when they had their first menstrual cycle, showed that girls with low levels of leptin in their bloodstreams reached puberty later than girls who had exceeded a certain threshold level of leptin. And while the evidence is less clear, leptin may also be linked to a delay in puberty in boys. Research has shown that leptin levels often peak right before the initiation of puberty in young men, implying that the peak is somehow involved in signaling the body to begin its change to adulthood.

Of course, a starving animal's most immediate need is to find food, and leptin is involved in jump starting this process too. A drop in leptin boosts the levels of the handful of chemicals floating around in our brains that compel us to eat. Sarah Leibowitz, a neurobiologist at Rockefeller University, has spent the last decade studying such neurochemicals. She has focused on a substance known as neuropeptide Y, or NPY—one of the most effective eating stimulants ever found. According to Leibowitz, NPY is particularly adept at making us crave carbohydrates. The more NPY our brains produce, the more carbohydrates we eat.

As Leibowitz points out, when our bodies get less food because we're on a diet, it is no different from eating less because the hunt was unsuccessful or a jackal ate the tribe's food supply. While a dieter may reduce his or her food consumption only slightly, an insufficient number of calories is enough to make the body think that it is being deprived. Therefore, people who try to lose weight by fasting or skipping meals are, says Leibowitz, doomed from the start. Dieting upsets the natural daily rhythms of the neurochemicals that control appetite. It sends NPY levels through the roof, guaranteeing that when the next mealtime comes around we will be ravenous. And the same compounds that affect appetite also affect mood, state of mind, and how energetic we feel. Mild degrees of food restriction, like missing a meal, have been associated with impairments in short-term memory, in sustained attention, in reaction times, and in spatial reasoning.

"Faking" Out the Body

Determined to find a way to fool the body into thinking it is eating when it's not, many people have turned to artificial sweeteners. Yet researchers say that whether you're partial to the little pink packets or to the blue ones, to Tab or Diet Coke, this kind of dietary sleight of hand is generally a waste of time. Our bodies' enormous sensitivity to not only how many calories we eat but also what form the calories take is one reason why the dietetic foods boom has failed to have an impact on our national waistline.

Researchers studying the effects of artificial sweeteners on our eating habits and our ability to lose weight have found that diet foods may alter the types of foods we eat—people may substitute carbohydrates like sugar for fats, for example. But overall they have no net effect on the number of calories we take in, and therefore they have no net effect on weight.

When test subjects aren't told anything about the snacks they are given, their bodies do an extraordinary job of regulating the number of calories they ingest over the course of a day. Subjects given snacks that are sweetened with real sugar compensate by eating fewer calories at the following meal. In contrast, people who eat snacks that are sweetened with artificial sweeteners like aspartame (as in NutraSweet) eat just as much at the following meal as subjects whose snacks are left unsweetened. Which means that fake sugars don't fool your body into thinking that it has eaten sugary foods.

Now that may not be the point for some people. They may choose a diet soda solely so that they can get their calories from dessert rather than from their soft drink. But it isn't going to help them lose weight because the body knows exactly how many carbohydrates it is eating, and it regulates that intake fairly closely. Protein is even more closely monitored. When either nutrient is eaten to excess, the body simultaneously burns more of it and suppresses our appetite for it at subsequent meals, which is one of the reasons high-protein diets are so effective at squelching appetite.

However, fat seems to be less clearly regulated than proteins or carbohydrates. Fat in foods triggers the release of biochemical signals that suppress hunger, just as carbohydrates and proteins do. Yet the body fails to put on the brakes for fat as effectively as it does for these other nutrients. Instead of responding by immediately burning more fat, the body reacts in a roundabout way. It gradually increases fat stores. More fat storage means that more free-floating fat becomes available in the bloodstream as fuel. Eventually this has the effect of boosting the rate at which fat is burned. But compared to the control mechanisms for proteins and carbohydrates, the effect is both subtle and indirect.

It's not clear why fat is the weakest of the nutrients in suppressing subsequent intake. Some researchers have suggested that the brakes on fat consumption were never designed to cope with the amount of fat currently in the western diet. But regardless of why, the fact that the body doesn't regulate fat intake very well means that when we eat a high-fat diet, we usually wind up eating more calories than we need. It has also led to the hope that, unlike artificial sweeteners, fake fats may be able to slide in under the body's radar, thus decreasing the overall calories that people consume and helping them to lose weight.

In January 1996, the FDA approved olestra—the first new nutrient to enter the food supply since the sweetener aspartame was approved in 1981. Olestra was discovered in the late 1960s by Procter & Gamble scientists who were trying to find a substance that premature babies could readily digest. In the process they created a fat that, because of its unusual chemical structure, people could not digest. Thirty-odd years and a lot of tinkering later, the company's food engineers produced a product with all the taste, smell and mouthfeel of real fat but none of the calories, which would seem to make it the product we have all been waiting for—except for a few drawbacks.

Olestra, which is synthesized from molecules of sugar and vegetable oil, depletes the body of the fat-soluble vitamins A, D, E, and K. Foods containing olestra must be supplemented with these vitamins. More important, olestra drags carotenoids out of the body—compounds that give fruits and vegetables their red, orange or yellow color and have been shown to lower the risk of cancer and heart disease. Many people have probably heard of beta carotene and the recent debate over whether supplementing our diets with it is beneficial. There are about 500 carotenoids in nature, and our understanding of how all these substances work in the body is sketchy enough to make supplementing olestra foods with them an impossible task. Procter & Gamble's argument that most people won't be eating olestra snacks during regular meals—the times when they would generally be eating carotenoid-containing fruits and vegetables—provides little comfort.

The most disturbing aspect of olestra, however, and the one for which it is most renowned, is really rather disgusting. During the early days of product testing, Procter & Gamble gave volunteers who had eaten olestra a questionnaire to fill out that included pictures of stained underwear on a graded scale from one to eight. The testers were asked to rank the extent of their gastrointestinal disturbance by choosing the underwear that most closely resembled their own. "And let me tell you, eight was a wow!" says Myra Karstadt, a senior scientist with the Center for Science in the Public Interest, who reviewed Procter & Gamble's research on olestra. Since then, the fake fat has been tinkered with to make it less leak-induc-ing. But not enough to spare olestra products from the FDA requirement that they carry a warning label: "Olestra may cause abdominal cramping and loose stools."

If olestra's nutritional and gastrointestinal effects aren't enough to give you pause, there is still the issue of effectiveness. Whether or not this indigestible fat will live up to its suggestive new name—Procter & Gamble has renamed it Olean—is still an open question. Researchers at Pennsylvania State University, in collaboration with Procter & Gamble, found that substituting olestra chips for regular chips did decrease the average number of calo-ries and percentage of fat that participants in the study ate. But this was true only for the people who didn't know that olestra had been substituted for the fat in the chips they were served. The result hints at the much trickier issue of how people deal with food in the real world.

Numerous studies have shown that if people are told they are being given food that is low-cal (whether or not it actually is), they will eat more at the next meal than peo-ple who are given the same food but told that it is full of calories. Mentally the ones who think they're eating diet food give themselves permission to pig out the rest of the day. Most of these studies have been done with artificially sweetened food, but the results are the same for low-fat foods. In the Pennsylvania study, the people who knew they were eating olestra chips ate enough extra calories to make up for the ones they had missed. Researchers now call this phenomenon the Snackwells effect. If a cookie is labeled fat-free, why not have two, or the whole box?

It may take a few chip-laden Super Bowl Sundays before we know the true outcome of olestra's market launch. But if this artificial fat helps people eat fewer calories only when they don't know they're eating it, then that defeats the purpose, since products that contain olestra clearly state that on the label. Even if you manage to trick someone into eating these chips without knowing the contents (a possibility, since they look and taste pretty much like ordinary chips), that person may still get the message in the form of gastric distress.

Then again, maybe not. Olestra seems to sail through some people's bodies most of the time. Finding out whether you are one of those people merely means stepping up to the olestra slot machine and taking a chance on diarrhea and a few other nasty effects. Hey, it all might be worth it for the chance to eat chips to your heart's content. In fact, all our efforts at dieting might be considered harmless jousting with our bodies' defenses were it not for the fact that this thrust and parry can have disastrous effects.

Dieting Ruins Nature

Obesity researchers have long been aware that stringent dieting is a major trigger for binge eating. The classic study proving this connection was done during World War II by University of Minnesota physiologist Ancel Keys. In 1944 Keys recruited three dozen conscientious objectors for a study on the effects of starvation. He put this group of young healthy men on a diet that consisted of about half the number of calories they were used to eating. Keys referred to the diet as semistarvation but, truth be told, it was not much different from the kinds of diets people are routinely put on by commercial weight loss programs.

For six months, the men dedicated themselves to this dietary regime with religious devotion. They dropped massive amounts of weight. But the effort took its toll. The men became glum and lethargic. They snapped at one another frequently. In Keys's analysis of the study, he writes of their "depression" and "emotional instability." Dieting had put them into a completely different mindset, familiar to anyone who has tried a semistarvation diet.

What's more, as soon as Keys freed the men to eat what they wanted, they went on massive eating binges. They gorged themselves for weeks, yet still reported gnawing feelings of hunger. Their weight came back on quickly, but most of the men completely lost the muscle tone they once had. The new weight was mainly fat. Only once they had returned to their normal weight, plus a little more for most of the men, did their foul moods and their lethargy finally dissipate.

Keys's study is one of many that University of Toronto psychologist Janet Polivy points to when she says that dieting is the main source of the compulsive eating that plagues so many people. Polivy, who has studied dieting for the last 25 years, believes people rarely get fat by going on binges but instead binge because they have been depriving themselves on a restrictive diet.

The effects of deprivation go deep. Besides causing people to gain back the weight they may have lost, and often a few extra pounds, dieting teaches people to ignore the natural signals their bodies use to express hunger and satiety, according to Polivy. The result is that once people go off a diet they have no idea how to eat normally. The natural tendency of their bodies to return to set-point becomes a vicious cycle in which they try to overrule natural signals. Instead of relying on internal cues such as hunger, they let their minds decide when and what it is okay to eat.

Without realizing it, they are setting themselves up for failure. The biochemical signals that tell us we are satisfied are affected not only by how much we eat but by what foods we eat. If you crave ice cream, a carrot stick just won't do. Everybody knows the feeling of being gastronomically unsatisfied. Unless you feed your body what it wants, you end up feeling deprived and, in many cases, eating more in the long run. Instead of getting thinner, dieters may see their weight moving steadily skyward.

Inevitably they will spend more and more of their energy thinking about food. Keys's starving conscientious objectors bear this out. During the six months they were kept on a low-calorie diet, they spent hours thinking, dreaming, and talking of food—fabulous dishes they would have once the diet ceased. They lost interest in cultural events, in sex. They hung pictures of food on their walls. A couple even made plans to become chefs.

Polivy has seen the same preoccupation with food in many lifelong dieters. These so-called restrained eaters are perpetually depriving themselves, causing their brains to divert much of their energy toward securing food.

Naturally their thoughts turn to eating. They are more likely to tell you what they had for dinner than who they ate it with. They may remember social occasions not by the calendar date or even the mood of the event but by what was served.

Gwen Shamblin refers to such people as having a "love affair with food." Yet according to Polivy it is no more than an obsession that is born of attempts to diet. Rather than shameful gluttony, it is a situation that has been thrust on them because of the conflict between a culture that tells them to pursue thinness and a biology that resists this directive.

Such an obsession affects Kay (not her real name), a woman who went through one of Gwen Shamblin's Weigh Down Workshops. Asked what brings her joy in life, she says, "a plate of fettucini." She has seen her weight as a problem ever since she reached puberty, and it has climbed in fits and starts ever since. She lost 50 pounds for a high school reunion, then put them back on with the birth of her first child. A glamour shot of her in a negligee hangs on one of the walls in her bedroom and at different times in her life, depending on her weight, she has looked at it and thought that she was either terribly fat in the picture or impressively svelte.

One day an article about Shamblin's diet program appeared in her local newspaper. "I decided I hadn't wasted good money on disappointing, temporary weight-loss efforts in quite a while," she says, "so I signed up." She dutifully attended Saturday afternoon classes where she "read a lot of Scripture" and watched Shamblin's video tapes. She found inspiration in the testimonials from program participants, along with before and after pictures showing some astounding weight losses. During the week between classes she listened to audio tapes.

Kay found Shamblin's tapes a bit amateurish. "She often pauses because she messed up a word or lost her train of thought and has to go back," says Kay. "But it kind of gives her a down-to-earth, sisterhood type of flavor." As for filling out the Weigh Down workbook, "thinking of different ways to glorify God in my life and writing prayer lists are a little bit of a stretch for me." She mainly read Shamblin's book.

Yet Kay claims just enough religious faith for Shamblin's message to strike a chord with her. "We don't go to church all that often," she says. "I don't pray every day. I just try to live like a good Christian. But then if somebody asks me, do I believe in God, I say, 'Hell, yes, I do!' So [Shamblin] puts you in a position where if you're saying 'I believe,' she makes you feel guilty into following."

Beyond Dieting

What Kay found in the midst of this wrapping of guilt was a program that conforms in a surprising number of ways to the antidieting advice of researchers like Polivy. The rules the Weigh Down Diet asked Kay to follow are based on sound physiological principles. In this respect, Shamblin has arrived in a somewhat circuitous manner at the same conclusions that many scientists have about the best way to take care of your weight, your body, and your health.

Whether you're talking about respecting your body because He gave it to you, because it is the only one you have, or because it is the product of millions of years of evolutionary history that have turned its weight-regulating system into a well-oiled machine, the upshot is still the same. Eat when you are hungry. Eat what you are hungry for. Stop when you are full. These are the tenets of the nondieting philosophy that both Shamblin and Polivy independently recommend.

They are a journey back to the days of unfettered eating that most of us experienced as infants and toddlers. At these tender ages, many studies have shown, children naturally know what foods they need to eat. Over a week's time, they will choose a balanced diet with all the required nutrients without anyone telling them how. But for some reason many of us lose the ability to do that when we become adults. We begin to rely on external cues, like the time of day or the size of our plate, to tell us when, what, and how much we need to eat.

That's why researchers like Polivy emphasize a nondieting approach as the only way to get past the crazed relationship with food that is so strongly enforced by our get-thin-quick culture. Contrary to what most people think, she says the best way to stop overeating is to stop dieting. The byproduct of this is that people will get back to a healthy, nonobsessive relationship with food, and their bodies will level off at their "natural" weights. But in order to reach that goal, people have to make some drastic changes in their lives. They may have to stop obsessing about being thin, accept their bodies for what they are, stop looking to food for entertainment, or quit using it to fill an emotional void.

In the case of Shamblin's program, all this is accomplished by putting control of weight in the hands of God and letting him be the one to dictate what the body needs—a prospect that is trickier than it sounds. "It's funny, because they lull you into thinking it's easy," says Kay, reflecting on her Weigh Down experience, "but you have to give up so much more. In other diet programs you have to weigh everything, so eating is a lot of work. In this it's nothing, no paperwork. This one is all about obedience. It's the most unusual thing I've ever experienced."

As it turns out, the task is both unusual and extraordinarily hard, whether it is giving control to God or just letting nature take its course. As Andria Siegler, a private counselor in Toronto, wrote in an essay entitled *Grieving the Lost Dreams of Thinness*, "Giving up dieting, especially for fat women, is not without consequences, for it can be synonymous with letting go of the dream, the hope, the fantasy of someday living life as a thin person. . . . The 'thinness package' usually contains any number of positive attributes, such as beauty, good health, success, glamour, fitness, intelligence, acceptance, sexiness, and of course, a mutually satisfying long-term love relationship! It is the perceived loss of the dream of this 'package,' not thinness per se, that is mourned so deeply by those becoming nondieters."

Siegler is a counselor for Beyond Dieting, one of the many secular nondieting programs that have risen, phoenix-like, from the more traditional approaches to

weight control and their long record of failure. Its goals
are not only to help people establish normal eating patterns but also to deal with the psychological consequences
of that choice. Women who go through the Beyond
Dieting program, says Siegler, often go through a grieving
process, the stages of which include frustration, envy, and
anger at the idea that some people can be thin without a
struggle while they cannot.

"It's a process that doesn't take place overnight," says
Cheri Erdman, a professor and counselor at the College of
DuPage in Glen Ellyn, Illinois, who did her dissertation on
women who had stopped dieting. She interviewed 18
women in the Chicago area and asked them two questions. Tell me your weight history. Tell me about when you
decided to stop dieting and just get on with your life.
Those who had entered the acceptance phase, she says,
were people who not only had a realistic body image but
had creatively attached to the idea of largeness some positive qualities, such as power and strength. These people
had also passed the stage of dividing their life into the
times when they were and were not thin. And most of the
women who got support from others in the early stages of
their move beyond dieting in later stages gave support.
Erdman found that it was important that these women
were "involved in something larger than themselves," a
statement that resonates with the approach of the Weigh
Down program.

Erdman is herself a former dieter, and she vividly
remembers the day she let go of her own dream of thinness. She had been exercising regularly for several years,

feeling healthy, and not worrying about her weight. "I remember going to the Y, swimming my laps, and feeling self-righteous. And I made the mistake of going on the scales. Of course I was over 200 pounds." That fact, staring her in the face despite all her efforts toward fitness drove her to tears. But then, she says, she had a realization: "My body has a mind of its own."

Erdman has now been a lap swimmer for over 15 years. Her cholesterol, blood pressure and other vital signs are normal and healthy. She boasts about her "athlete's pulse." And over the last six or eight years her weight has stabilized. Yet in telling her own story, Erdman makes an important point: giving up dieting isn't necessarily the road to weight loss.

To go from seeing food as either good or bad to feeding on demand is an enormous step for people who have spent most of their lives monitoring their food intake carefully. During the early stages of learning to hear what your body tells you, the possibility of eating what you want when you want is akin to letting a kid loose in a candy store. The first impulse is to eat everything in sight, and then eat some more. Eventually the attraction wears off, but what happens with your weight isn't known until it happens.

Experience with Beyond Dieting has shown that you might lose weight on such a program or you might not. Someone's natural weight may very well be the weight at which they started the program. If they are particularly restrained eaters—depriving themselves continually—

then their natural weight may be even higher. At the very least, people have to be willing to gain weight while they normalize their eating patterns. In fact, Donna Ciliska, one of the founders of the Beyond Dieting program, clearly states that it is not a weight loss program. The main idea of the Beyond Dieting program is to give up weight as a goal and accept health in its place.

This is a lesson that Gwen Shamblin has not yet taken to heart. Shamblin bends over backward to say that her program is a diet only in the sense that the word means the food and drink you regularly consume, as opposed to a strict, prescribed eating plan. She says that her publisher, Doubleday, insisted on using the word "diet" in the title of her book so that it would be shelved with books on diet and nutrition instead of in the religion or self-help sections. But the Weigh Down part of the name gives away the real goal; it is as a weight-loss program that it is pitched.

In the end, Shamblin still subscribes to the popular but limited view that fat is disgusting. During the studio taping session, she came up with the idea of passing around a piece of paper and asking everyone in the audience to write down how much weight they had lost. "Then we can videotape you all," she said, "and say something like, 'The floor says thank you!'"

One might think that the floor's feelings would be less important than those of some of the people in the audience who were still heavy and might feel criticized for burdening the floor with their excess weight. "The motivation to be thin is not vanity—it is natural," she writes in her book. "God has programmed us to want the best for our bodies."

Most of Shamblin's followers are as wrapped up in hating their fat as she is. That has been the wellspring of her program's ever-increasing appeal, as it is with all diet programs. But in riding the wave of obsession that fuels the diet advice industry in this country, Shamblin and other weight-loss gurus are doing a grave disservice to their followers. Thinness is a false God. One of the basic tenets of Christianity is that God loves all his children, the size sixteens no less than the size sixes. It is a philosophy to which we could all aspire.

Erdman's recollections of her own struggle with the dream of thinness bring up one final point worth emphasizing: Her weight stabilized with a regular program of exercise. Physical activity is something many dieters either ignore or approach with intense weight consciousness. As one former exercise addict confessed, "It started very simply for me. One mile equaled a hundred calories, so four miles equaled a milkshake. Before I knew it I was running marathons."

Such comments shed light on one of the main reasons that even weight maintenance programs like Beyond Dieting have tended to treat exercise with kid gloves: people can be as obsessive about exercising to lose weight as they can be about dieting. Even if, intellectually, people know that stress relief, strength, enhanced creativity, and long life are among the many benefits of physical activity, it is still extremely difficult for them to drop the idea that the only reason to exercise is to take off weight. Yet this lack of emphasis on activity as a natural part of everyone's life is an extraordinary oversight. Not only is exercise one of the few things that have been shown to promote long-term weight stability; it is the routine maintenance that keeps our bodies and our minds running smoothly.

FOUR

The Successful Loser

HOW EXERCISE AFFECTS BODY AND MIND

Marisol Dominguez emerges from a shower stall dripping wet. A pair of shorts made of hospital-gown material clings to her hips. She pads across a tile floor in beige foam slippers and climbs a short stepladder up the side of a small concrete tank that has been specially designed to measure underwater weight. "Mmm, warm water. I love it," she says, slipping her leg into the greenish pool and then crouching inside. To Dominguez, this is all a familiar routine. She first encountered the tank two years ago, in the Body Composition Lab at St. Luke's–Roosevelt Hospital in Manhattan. She was just about to begin a weight-loss program. Now, having lost the weight, she is back for a follow-up visit.

"Okay, now let's go through the test again just in case you don't remember," says Albert Kovera, a graduate student in the lab. He recites a set of instructions with the rhythm of a practiced speech. "What you're going to do is you're going to grab onto both sides of the silver bar at the bottom, and while your head is above water you're going to take in a big deep breath. A really exaggerated breath. Whoooo," he demonstrates. "Then you just blow out hard and fast. Keep blowing and blowing all that air out until you feel like you can't get anything else out of your lungs, seal your lips, then dunk yourself underwater."

It's like asking someone to keep a finger in a flame when every fiber of their being is telling them to pull it away. Dominguez has to overcome a strong survival instinct in order to submerge herself after giving up all her air. She comes up sputtering the first time. Her will to live gets the better of her and she takes a quick breath at the last second, making water go up her nose. Once again she goes down. She has to wait underwater until Kovera knocks on the side of the tank. He tells her it will only be about three seconds; it is seven.

While Dominguez crouches underwater, Kovera stares at a machine that looks like a miniature polygraph. Its pen moves back and forth across a sheet of paper—the midpoint of this zigzag is Dominguez's underwater weight. Several dunks later, Kovera takes an average of the midpoints, 4.3 kilograms, then moves across the room to enter it into a computer. From this figure the computer can generate the most accurate assessment currently available of a body's density. It then uses this number to calculate the body's percentage of fat. Dominguez's is 17 percent. That's low. Average is about 25 percent, Kovera says. A female body builder who once came into the lab had 8.8 percent body fat. Women don't get much leaner than that.

Dominguez has her street clothes on and her hair toweled dry by the time Kovera has finished calculating her internal information. She walks out of the Body Composition Lab through a maze of basement hallways, shunning the elevator in favor of two flights of stairs. Outside, on East 116th Street, the sun is bright. Dominguez's damp arms dart and glint as she begins to fill me in on her weight-loss saga. Six years ago she was over 210 pounds. Now she weighs 138. "I have a photograph," she says. "Do you want to see it?"

I ask her if she always carries a picture of her former self. "No, I actually found it the other day to show it to somebody." A truck speeds past and she shouts to be heard above the din. I struggle to project Dominguez's kinetic personality onto the woman in the photograph. Even her face bears only a faint resemblance, like a cousin or a sister. The transformation is incredible.

Dominguez's is the kind of achievement that nearly every heavy person holds in the back of the mind. She was fat once, and now she is lean. She set her mind to the task, and then she accomplished it. Stories of people like Dominguez dropping massive amounts of weight are not uncommon. There are enough of them to fuel an entire diet industry full of before and after shots. But in Dominguez's case the weight has stayed off, and that is an anomaly. How did she do it? How does anyone do it?

The Registry

During a conversation obesity researcher James Hill, at the University of Colorado Health Sciences Center in Denver, was having with his colleague Rena Wing, at the University of Pittsburgh School of Medicine, they kept running up against the fact that everything they knew about weight loss had come from people who ultimately failed at it. The vast majority of people who lose weight regain one-third to two-thirds of it within a year, and almost all of it by five years.

This was the conclusion drawn by an NIH Technology Assessment Conference Panel that met in the spring of 1992 and published its findings the following year. The panel combined the results of a handful of scientific studies that evaluated dietary success rates to arrive at its statement. But because of this approach, Hill and Wing, like a number of other obesity researchers, suspected that the panel's conclusion was grimmer than reality.

Not only are there relatively few such studies, but they are often of short duration and can have dropout rates as high as 80 percent. In most of these studies, the results reflect weight loss from diet alone, not diet with exercise and/or behavior modification. Most important, such studies take place in clinical settings, which means that their results don't necessarily reflect the success of average dieters.

The majority of people who are trying to lose weight never go to a doctor or a weight-loss specialist. Most of them don't even enter commercial weight-loss programs.

Instead, 95 percent of men and 87 percent of women glean information from popular books and magazines and then design their own eating and exercise regimen.

If they are successful—well, they get lost between the cracks. Most people know someone who needed to lose 20 or 30 or 40 pounds. The person decided one day to do something about it and then did, without ever being studied by scientists. Any reasonable estimate of how many people successfully lose weight and keep it off has to include this hidden group.

A somewhat unscientific survey may provide the best available estimate for how well average people maintain a weight drop. In 1993 Consumer Reports magazine asked 95,000 of its readers about the success of their diets. The results of the poll showed that of the respondents who had lost weight, 30 percent of them kept off more than two-thirds of it after two years.

So even though Hill called it hopeful thinking, he and Wing were probably justified in their assumption that the number of people who manage to lose weight and keep it off is higher than the NIH panel implied. "We thought, wouldn't it be interesting to look at some people who succeeded," says Hill. And armed with this idea, he and Wing set out to look for that rare and oxymoronic creature, the successful loser.

They contacted the Sandoz Corporation, makers of Optifast (the liquid diet program that Oprah Winfrey used a few years ago to shed 67 pounds), and asked if they could send a letter to the company's clients asking those people who had lost weight and kept it off if they would like to join a National Weight Control Registry. A few names trickled in. The occasional newspaper article prompted more. Then *Parade* magazine, which has a circulation of 37 million, ran an article and the project snowballed. The size of the registry more than tripled, as 2500 new people wrote in. With these kinds of numbers, Hill and Wing began to think they were finally onto something.

If you ask any individual how he or she lost weight, you'll get a personal story. Dominguez, for example, had some food sensitivities and was somewhat lactose intolerant, so when she started her weight-loss program her diet became a kind of research project. She pored over the diet and fitness books that were out on the market. She looked at vitamin manuals. She didn't take every word they said literally, she just picked the things that made sense to her. She lost 65 pounds in the first six months and plateaued there for over a year. Then she went through the weight-loss program at St. Luke's to drop the last few pounds.

But while her technique and her success might be enough to get her a contract deal to write her own diet book, such personal stories aren't very helpful to researchers trying to advise people on how to take off weight. One woman's successful technique won't necessarily work for anybody else, particularly over the long term. That's where the registry differs. By looking at the techniques and stories of hundreds of people, Hill and Wing hope to find some common truths about what works and about what happens to your body when it undergoes such a dramatic weight change.

Hill has just the tool to make that happen. A short walk from his office in the heart of Denver is a neatly appointed room just a little bigger than a household bathroom. In it, there is a desk, a futon, and a small window. On a clear day you can see Pike's Peak in the distance. But it's not for the luxury accommodations that people come to this room. One day in here and Hill can tell you precisely how much energy you expended every minute of your stay just by looking at the oxygen you consumed and the carbon dioxide you produced. He can also tell you exactly what kinds of calories you burned—fat, protein, or carbohydrates. These are just the kinds of details Hill would like to know about his registry members, which is why he will be flying some of them in to do 24-hour stints in the calorimetry chamber.

Inside this tiny box, under the constant watch of technicians, they'll recreate the kind of activity they would do on a normal day. One veteran of the chamber, a fit-looking man named Jay, who spent five separate nights in the room for a study on exercise, claims that the task is easier than you might think. "You call people up. There's a TV. I took some paperwork. It really went by very fast." A couple of study subjects have brought in Nintendo sets. One native American medical student passed the time making a beaded quiver for his future in-laws. Only one person has ever had to come out during a study, according to Teresa Sharp, the chamber's designer and caretaker, and that was because of a family emergency, not cabin fever. "Most people aren't as claustrophobic as you'd think," she says. "And anyway, we keep them pretty busy."

Because the chamber is so small, recreating an average day requires some elaborate choreography. Take a simple chore like going to the bathroom, for example. There is a toilet in the chamber, of course. But to duplicate the effort of walking down a hall or up a set of stairs to the bathroom, subjects have to pace back and forth for a carefully measured interval before they can actually sit down. The same sort of scrutiny applies to eating. Every meal contains a calculated number of calories. Study subjects have to eat the entire meal and spread it evenly over a 15-minute time period. Before and after they eat, they have to push a button that marks each event for the technicians collecting data outside the room. The hope is that this sort of painstaking information from registry participants will add up to much broader answers about their successful weight loss.

Insights from the Registry

"One of the things that we're interested in," says Hill, "is if you take people who have maintained their weight for only a year and people who have done it for ten years, do you begin to see that maybe the people that are ten years out are sort of metabolically normal, whereas the one-year people might show some metabolic changes that could cause weight regain? Which might allow us to say, look, there's some point in time at which, if you maintain, it actually becomes easier to maintain."

Even before the calorimetry studies and other metabolic tests are complete, some conclusions can be drawn from the answers registry members have given on a series of questionnaires. For instance, Hill says that one of the most interesting things about the registry is that these are people who have tried to lose weight previously and failed. Not only were they veteran dieters, but most had been overweight since childhood. That is heartening in a way. It means that even people who have been unable to lose weight in the past or unable to keep it off may be able to do so at some time in the future. But it also raises a question: What was it that allowed the registry members to succeed this time?

As Hill points out, "These people knew what to do before, when they were unsuccessful. It's not like they learned some secret that let them do it. It's more, this time they really had the motivation to do it." What motivated many of the men in the registry, the researchers have found, was a medical event—a heart attack, for example— that turned their struggle with weight into a choice between life and an early death. For women, the triggers were less consistent—an upcoming anniversary, physical discomfort, or just one too many comments about their weight. Regardless of the reason, these people all managed to find a resolve that had eluded them before.

Psychological assessments of the registrants using a variety of different tests reveal another commonality among the group. Even years after losing the weight, the registrants typically show higher levels of dietary restraint. Restraint is a term that obesity researchers use to indicate that someone is watching what they eat and in what portions. By and large, Hill says, the registrants aren't obsessed with weight and food, but they are careful about it. In other words they didn't lose the weight and then magically change into the kinds of people who eat what they want whenever they want it.

In fact, Hill has a special term for registry members that pretty well sums up their current status. He calls them the reduced obese. "I don't think the reduced obese ever go back to that level where they just really aren't concerned with food and activity patterns and so forth," he says. "I think they will always be concerned with it." Which lends credence to the idea that giving up dieting, while it may be the best remedy for food obsession, is not necessarily the road to weight loss.

The same conclusions Hill and Wing are drawing from their registrants are echoed in studies of weight control in monkeys. Barbara Hansen, the director of the Obesity Research Center at the University of Maryland School of Medicine, once forced a group of monkeys to lose weight by putting them on a diet. She then kept them at a reduced weight for two years, "on the idea that maybe you could habituate them to eat a different amount of calories," she explained one day from her Baltimore office. A silence filled the telephone line as Hansen paused here for effect, then let out a hearty "Hah! The minute we allowed them to free feed, they regained their weight at exactly the same rate as another group of monkeys that had been weight-reduced for only three months. So there was no resetting of the animals' set-points and no fixing of their behavior based on two years of a diet that kept them stable in weight." Like the registry's reduced obese, the monkeys' weight maintenance was solely the result of restraint, though in this case the willpower was supplied by their caretakers.

Dominguez seemed to follow this pattern as well. Though I didn't spend enough time with her to say whether she is a restrained eater, it was clear from our short conversation on 116th Street that she still has a centurion's vigilance about what goes into her body. "I'm taking my vitamins and eating vegetables or fruits—high priority," she says at the start of a spontaneous diatribe. "I don't care who says I can't have lentil beans. Eat something. Eat some broccoli, eat some spinach, eat some kale, eat some cauliflower. You need your greens. You need your C. You need your D. You need your E. You need protein. If you can't have meat, eat your beans. You need some protein. Oatmeal is protein."

If she seems a touch preoccupied with her eating, she is positively possessed when the conversation turns to exercise. She was wearing sweats the day I met her, and from the sound of it this has been her uniform for the last two years. When she began her weight-loss program she was in the gym seven days a week, usually twice a day. She often went in at noon, worked out for an hour, broke for lunch and errands and then went back to the gym for another hour and a half. She'd split her routines—do stationary bike in the morning, weights in the afternoon. Some days her pace would be moderate, other days intense. "I wouldn't suggest the way I was working," she says. "It was kind of radical."

But she is still working out almost daily, and this sort of major commitment to activity, Hill says, is the common denominator for virtually all the people in the registry. They increased their physical activity enormously. On average they report expending 2,829 calories a week through physical activity. That's roughly the equivalent of six and a half hours of jogging. It is widely acknowledged by exercise physiologists that when people are surveyed about how much they exercise, they often overestimate. But even if these are exaggerated activity estimates, Hill says, these people are still working out a tremendous amount. By and large, they're doing the kinds of activities they don't consider torture. For women, that generally means walking or aerobics. The men tend toward lifting weights or participating in sports. Hill ascribes most of the weight loss and maintenance to this one key change in their lifestyles.

How Exercise Helps People Lose Weight

There are several ways exercise may help people take off and keep off weight—most of which are familiar to anyone who has struggled with dropping a few extra pounds. The first and most obvious way is that while you are exercising, your body burns more calories. It has to provide energy to the contracting muscles. The energy comes from burning the carbohydrates, fats, and proteins you have eaten. During exercise, the body's need for energy can be 10 to 15 times what it is at rest.

In addition to the calories burned during an exercise like jogging, your overall metabolism is cranked up for some time after you hop off the treadmill. Your body keeps burning energy at an elevated rate while it carries out the tasks of restoring its fuel reserves and building up the muscles you have been flexing. Even after all this work is complete, some of the hormones that were triggered by the exercise continue to float around in your body, keeping metabolism high, until they gradually degrade.

How long enhanced metabolism continues depends on the intensity and duration of the exercise—more exercise has greater effects. When you increase the amount of muscle in your body, you may also experience a subtle but significant rise in your long-term metabolic rate, because muscle tissue uses more calories on a day-to-day basis than fat does. Researchers disagree on the level of training required to get this overall boost in metabolism, and the benefits may go only to those who do high-intensity workouts.

Exercise also increases your appetite, and that leads many dieters to worry that they are wasting their time by working out. But the heightened desire to eat doesn't make up for the extra energy used by exercising, at least at the beginning of an exercise program. Later, after your body has settled into a new level of physical activity, it takes in the number of calories it needs to keep your weight on an even keel. But by then, your weight may already be lower. And even if you stay the same weight, you look thinner when you are exercising, which for some people may be the most important reason to do it. A pound of muscle takes up less space than a pound of fat.

Of all the weight-loss techniques that have been tried over the years, exercise is the only one that has consistently been shown to help people keep weight off. This is true whether or not people are dieting. In fact, a program of regular exercise without dieting may be the best strategy of all for long-term weight maintenance.

Recently John Foreyt's lab, at the Baylor College of Medicine in Houston, performed a study on three groups of people: volunteers who dieted only, those who dieted and exercised, and those who exercised only. You might think that the diet-plus-exercise group lost the most weight—diet plus exercise beats either diet or exercise alone in most studies—and after a year that was true. The diet-plus-exercise group lost an average of 20 pounds each, compared to 15 pounds for the diet-only group and 6 for those who exercised only. But by the end of the second year of the study, the tables had turned. The exercise-only group kept off all but 1 of the pounds they had lost. The dieters regained 17 pounds, leaving them 2 pounds heavier than when they started, and the diet and exercisers regained 15 pounds.

The probable cause for these results given by the researchers was that dieting is just extremely hard to keep up over the years. And often when people blow their diets, they go overboard and eat as if there were no tomorrow. Exercise produced smaller weight losses, but it proved to be a better long-term strategy, which brings up an important point about exercise: its benefits may be more than the sum of the calories it burns.

Kelly Brownell, a psychologist and director of the Yale Center for Eating and Weight Disorders, speculates that the effect of exercise on weight control cannot be explained by physiological effects alone. He claims that psychological factors will be shown to explain more of the variance in weight control than will physiological factors.

Most dieters know that it is much easier to cut calories by eating fewer than by trying to exercise them off. In fact, true weight-loss mavens can usually rattle off the exact number of calories burned by their preferred form of activity. Susan, a Virginia resident who has a treadmill in her basement, clocks her daily workout time by what she had for lunch. A cheeseburger equals about an hour on the treadmill. A salad buys her a break.

Yet in spite of how much work it takes to burn a few dozen calories, regular exercise is the strongest predictor of whether someone will lose weight and maintain the loss. "This," Brownell points out, "suggests some nonbiological factor as the mechanism." Somehow exercise influences our thoughts and our feelings in a way that, in turn, influences our ability to eat less or eat better.

Brownell also says that based on observations of his own patients, many people who exercise and maintain weight losses are doing the kind of low-intensity activities (for example, walking or gardening) that aren't likely to have strong effects on their metabolic rates. They would have to be doing a lot of gardening to explain the weight loss in terms of the calories burned. Finally, Brownell points to the vast array of evidence that exercise has impressive psychological benefits.

For example, in one study in which obese people were tested and then reexamined four years later, exercise corresponded with improved well-being, improved eating self-efficacy, and lower depression for both test years. Other studies have shown conflicting results when it comes to depression. For example, while exercise clearly can reduce depression in people who are moderately depressed to start out with, it doesn't always do so in normal populations. But dozens of other studies agree that exercise increases peoples' satisfaction with their lives and gives them a greater sense of control over their eating. It has also been shown to reduce stress and improve self-esteem.

What is still unclear is exactly how exercise effects these psychological changes. For example, does running improve our mood because it has some effect on endorphins or other aspects of our body chemistry? Or is the mere act of doing something positive for our bodies enough to cheer us up? The answer is somewhat important, according to Brownell, because if it's just a matter of biochemistry, then what we think about the exercise we're doing would have no effect on the final outcome.

If, on the other hand, the effects of exercise on weight control are more psychological than physiological, then what matters is what we define as a positive act. If we are convinced that only intense exercise "counts," then indeed we will have to do intense exercise to get a psychological lift. People either need to do the exercise they believe will help them, or they need to convince themselves that activities that may be less intense but more enjoyable, and therefore more likely to be continued, are equally beneficial.

By exploring such issues Brownell opens up a psychological door that few obesity researchers have entered. The vast majority of research that looks at why exercise helps people maintain their weight loss has focused on its metabolic effects. More important, it defines the benefits of exercise in terms of its effects on weight.

That thinking is largely a reflection of our weight-driven culture. In the minds of many dieters, exercise is synonymous with calorie burning, and for many athletes, weight control is their primary motivation. In a survey of over 4,000 readers of *Runner's World* magazine, Brownell and his colleagues found that 48 percent of the women and 21 percent of the men said that they were often, usually, or always "terrified of being fat."

But let's face it, exercise, despite all the weight benefits mentioned, doesn't make you thin automatically. The people in Foreyt's exercise-only study lost five pounds after four years, and that result is representative of most studies in which people boost their activity levels for a few hours a week. Only in studies of extensive exercise regimens—five months of basic military training, for example—do researchers see larger weight losses, and these average between 10 and 35 pounds.

The biggest effects of exercise for most people are not on weight but on health. At her peak weight, Dominguez says she could barely walk down the street. For her, the motivation not only to start working out but to continue long after the weight had fallen off was that she felt her health was in jeopardy. "I needed to do it for myself," she says, "not just to be cute and chic and thin."

Exercise May Be All You Really Need for Good Health

There are many reasons why people might want to be "normal" weight rather than obese. Constant harassment is just one of them. But consider the possibility that weight loss may take a backseat to activity in terms of what's really best for your body. In other words, the choice may not be fit or fat, as Covert Bailey would put it, but fit and fat. "Quite frankly, I think fitness is more important than obesity," says Steven Blair, an exercise physiologist at the Cooper Institute of Aerobics Research in Dallas. "It certainly is at least as important."

For over a quarter of a century, Blair and his colleagues have been keeping health statistics on a large group of men and women and looking at how physical activity and, perhaps more important, the lack of it affect the incidence of disease and death. In 1994 Blair was asked to speak at a meeting on exercise and obesity that was part of an international conference of obesity researchers in Quebec city. The invitation prompted him to look specifically at the obese people in his study group to see what role their weights and their activity levels had in causing their premature deaths.

All of Blair's study subjects underwent an initial fitness test. Blair put them on a treadmill and gradually increased the grade at which they were walking over the first 25 minutes of the test, then held the grade constant and gradually turned up the speed until the subjects were finally forced by exhaustion to quit. The length of time they managed to stay on the treadmill was a measure of their cardiorespiratory fitness. This figure correlates well with a more common measure of fitness, VO2max, which is the maximum amount of oxygen a person is able to use per minute, per kilogram of body weight, during a comparable stress test on a treadmill or exercise bike.

The problem with using either of these measurements to define someone's level of physical activity is that fitness depends not just on being active but also on genetic endowment. Some people naturally have a stronger cardiorespiratory system than others. They may score well on a stress test even though they are relatively sedentary. But since people generally become more fit as they increase their activity, fitness is at least a reasonable indicator of how sedentary or how active a person is. The main advantage of measuring fitness rather than asking people to report on their level of activity, Blair says, is that it can be objectively determined in the laboratory.

Blair's treadmill test thus allowed him to divide a group of 25,389 men of all weights into different fitness categories. Blair then looked closely at the 673 men who died during the 19-year run of the study. What he found went against the grain of what most people, and most obesity researchers, were thinking at that time. Obesity kills—that's been the standard line since population-wide studies began showing that obesity often correlates with an increased risk of premature death from a variety of diseases. Over the last half a dozen years, the word epidemic has come into fashion to describe what is already among the most loathed of human conditions. Yet Blair found that the most important factor in the premature deaths of these men was not how fat they were but how physically fit.

In fact all the men who were fit, whether they were obese, overweight, or normal weight, had roughly the same death rate—20 per 10,000 men over the course of the follow-up period. By comparison, the men who were unfit had death rates that were three times the "fit" rate. In the least fit obese men, 62 of every 10,000 men died. In the least fit lean men the rate was 52 per 10,000. Which means that normal-weight men who weren't fit were nearly three times as likely to die as the fat men who were fit. Blair's conclusion was clear: If living a long life is the objective, then it's better to be fat and fit than svelte and sedentary.

The fact is that the same people who fall into the category of obese in most population-wide surveys also tend to be less active, and thus less physically fit, than their leaner counterparts. "Given that we know that as a group fat people are more sedentary and unfit," Blair asks, "then when we see fat people dying at a higher rate than normal-weight people, how do we just automatically know that it's the obesity and not the inactivity that's causing the deaths? I raise that as a question to scientists. Well, how do you know?"

Perhaps it took a man of a certain stature to punch holes in the assumption that skinny equals healthy. Blair is himself quite stocky (as well as short and bald, he points out good-humoredly) but extremely physically fit. He has been running virtually every day for the last 30 years. The same tenacity has brought his research widespread attention, though some of his fellow researchers have been slow to embrace it.

After decades of seeing obesity as the enemy, they have been understandably reluctant to give up the idea. Not only does it alter their treatment strategy, but it forces them to come face to face with their own prejudices. At conferences, scientists still worry out loud that people will be getting the wrong message if they're told that it's okay to be fat. But as Glenn Gaesser, an exercise physiologist at the University of Virginia, points out, for years society has operated under the impression that as long as you are lean it's okay to be inactive. Somehow this message is easier for many researchers to accept. Yet the work of Blair and others has demonstrated that this message is dead wrong.

The summary of the research on people of all shapes, sizes, and degrees of health is that a fit and active way of life extends longevity. This is true regardless of your starting weight and regardless of whether you lose weight by increasing your activity. The simple fact is that there are few things you can do that positively affect as many systems and organs in the body as exercise.

Regular physical activity can improve insulin sensitivity and blood pressure. It can increase the level of good (HDL) cholesterol and reduce the levels of triglycerides, or fats, in the bloodstream. These are all indicators of our risk for diabetes, coronary heart disease, and other chronic and debilitating conditions. One of the many ways exercise provides these benefits is by boosting the amount of blood that flows through our veins.

It takes only a single, intense exercise session to boost the total volume of blood in our bodies. One study found that male long-distance runners have almost a liter more blood than their more sedentary peers. But you don't have to be a marathoner to get the effect. Twenty-four hours after a vigorous workout, blood volume will have increased by 10 percent.

To push the extra blood around, our hearts not only beat faster but pump more blood with each "lub-dub." All this makes our heart muscles stronger and more efficient, which means that they end up doing less work when we are at rest. Both fit and unfit people have about the same cardiac output when they are just sitting around. But since a conditioned heart pumps more blood per beat, it ends up pumping less often. The resting heart rates of athletes are about 20 percent lower than the rates of nonathletes, and the overall amount of work that a conditioned heart does at rest is about 25 percent less.

The extra blood flow during exercise provides the oxygen and nutrients consumed by our muscles and carries away the carbon dioxide and heat produced. It also increases the circulation of the immune cells that fight bacteria, viruses, and tumors, which helps explain why physically fit people get fewer colds and other respiratory infections than people who are not fit. In one study, David Nieman, a professor of health and exercise science at Appalachian State University in Boone, North Carolina, showed that women who walked 40 to 45 minutes five days a week had half as many days with cold symptoms as people who didn't walk. Since the effects on circulation diminish rapidly after you stop exercising, daily or at least frequent activity is the best medicine, according to Nieman. But these weren't grueling workouts. All these people did was walk. This raises a question that many have asked but few have been able to answer. Just how hard do you have to exercise to get health benefits?

Exercise Lite

On a sunny July day in 1996, Al Gore and his wife, Tipper, invited photographers, journalists, and the usual entourage of Secret Service agents to join them on the White House grounds for a healthy workout. Tipper wore running shoes, and Al, southern boy that he is, wore cowboy boots. This isn't the kind of footwear one usually associates with vigorous physical activity. That the vice president could do any kind of exercise that would improve his health in such shoes was largely the point of this photo op.

It coincided with the release of the surgeon general's report on physical activity. For the first time, rather than exhorting Americans to feel the burn or make their hearts race, this document simply attempted to nudge us toward just a little more walking, a bit more gardening, and a slew of other "moderate" activities that don't really seem like exercise. This new way of thinking about activity has come to be known as Exercise Lite.

What prompted the shift? One catalyst was that the old recommendations for high-intensity workouts weren't working. In spite of America's reputation as a nation of joggers, the truth is that what we do best is wear the gear. Sweat suits are today's leisure suits. Suburban shopping malls are filled with people wearing them, but few of us actually do the activities for which the gear was designed.

According to the U.S. Department of Health and Human Services, 54 percent of adults fall short of the goal of 30 minutes of light to moderate physical activity per day. Twenty-four percent of adults are completely sedentary, doing no physical activity at all for the last month. The least sedentary adults are in the West, with Oregonians being the most active; 35.7 percent of the people from that state report some regular form of exercise. The most sedentary adults are in the District of Columbia, where only 16 percent of the adults say they exercise regularly and 49.3 percent say they do no exercise at all. Among kids, the numbers are equally disturbing. Only 37 percent of teens nationwide report regular vigorous exercise of 20 minutes or more three times a week.

One of the reasons many people shy away from exercise is that they believe you have to work out at a certain intensity and duration to have any real benefits. Exercise physiologists have nurtured such thinking because in most of their research over the years, the emphasis was on measuring fitness. Within this paradigm lay the unspoken assumption that the people who were in the best shape would get the health benefits. And indeed, many studies have shown that a high-intensity aerobic workout does wonders for our hearts and lungs. That doesn't mean that less intense exercise isn't also beneficial.

Given the black-and-white nature of the public discussion, many people opted for the easy road—no activity at all. And despite what might be referred to as the Oprah Winfrey excuse—I'd do it if I had a personal trainer—a 1996 study by Rena Wing showed that neither the use of a personal trainer who called people regularly and met them at their home or office at scheduled times for a walk nor an incentive program in which subjects received lottery tickets for working out improved exercise adherence.

It has been estimated that as many as 250,000 deaths per year in the United States are attributable to a lack of regular physical activity.

America's staggering lack of exercise has prompted a wake-up call to the nation's health policy community. That and a slew of new research has forced them to rethink their activity recommendations. Once exercise physiologists finally began questioning their assumptions about fitness levels, they found that people might not have to put themselves through strenuous workouts to reap health benefits.

The evidence was laid out most convincingly in a set of guidelines that came out three years before the surgeon general's report. In 1993 the Centers for Disease Control and Prevention and the American College of Sports Medicine (CDC/ACSM) convened a panel of 20 of the nation's experts on health and fitness. Their charge was to develop a clear, concise public health message regarding physical activity. The centerpiece of their recommendations was for Americans to accumulate 30 minutes or more of moderate-intensity physical activity at least five, and preferably seven, days a week.

They defined moderate activity as the equivalent of walking at three to four miles per hour. Four miles an hour is roughly the brisk pace people use when they're in a hurry to go somewhere. Their arms are swinging and their breathing is a little heavy, but their stride falls short of racewalking. This was a fairly mild regimen that the panel was recommending to improve the health of the nation. It was a marked change from the allegiance to intense workouts that had been firmly entrenched since the running boom of the 1970s.

The best argument that moderate activity provides health benefits comes from large observational studies of groups of people over extended time periods. One such study is known as the Multiple Risk Factors Intervention Trial (MRFIT). The MRFIT was designed to test whether intensive intervention would result in decreased death rates from coronary heart disease. Since 1973 its director, University of Minnesota epidemiologist Arthur Leon, has been following the health status of more than 12,000 men at high risk for that disease. After 16 years of study, Leon found that men who reported an average of 23 minutes a day of leisure time physical activity were 22 percent less likely to die from any cause and 29 percent less likely to die from coronary heart disease than men who averaged five minutes a day. The most common activities these men were doing were lawn and garden work, walking, and home repairs.

Leon also found that the death rates of men who were extremely active weren't significantly lower than those of men who were merely moderately active. In this respect, Leon's results differ somewhat from those of other large studies. Most researchers have found that the benefits of exercise do go up as people increase the amount and intensity of the exercise they do. The benefits just don't accrue as rapidly, or they improve some health statistics but not others.

For example, John Duncan, an exercise physiologist at the Cooper Institute, put three groups of women on different exercise regimens. The first group strolled (low intensity), the second walked briskly (moderate intensity), and the third group power walked (high intensity). All groups walked the same distance. Women in all three groups saw roughly the same improvement in their cholesterol levels. By this measure, there was no significant advantage to high-intensity training. But in the same study, the vigorous exercisers showed the largest improvement in cardiorespiratory capacity. They trained harder, and their hearts and lungs showed the results with improved aerobic fitness.

Given the somewhat conflicting evidence, the CDC/ACSM panel of experts chose a middle ground. They emphasized the benefits of moderate activity since they felt that this was a message an extremely sedentary population might actually take to heart. They justified their health message with the statement that their conclusions were "the most reasonable interpretation of the currently available data."

Critics like Paul Williams, an exercise researcher at the Lawrence Berkeley National Laboratory, have argued that these recommendations gave people the wrong impression: that doing high-intensity exercise is a waste of time. The panelists did seem to imply that beyond a certain level of fitness, each extra mile logged or flight of stairs climbed provided fewer returns. But since moderate exercise is easier to adhere to than intense exercise, getting people to do a reasonable amount of activity at a reasonable level of exertion seems more important over the long run than having them strive for peak fitness. And in fact that logic has an odd precedent, since it applies to other risk factors. For example, smoking a pack of cigarettes a day is bad for you, but it's not as bad as smoking three packs a day.

What's more, researchers like Abby King at the Stanford University School of Medicine have shown that high-intensity exercise is not necessary for psychological benefits to occur. While there is still some controversy over just how much and what intensity of activity is best, the basic message is clear: Do some. Do as much as you can manage and a range of health benefits will accrue.

Does all this mean that you can race the kids up the stairs to their bedrooms, tuck them in, then run downstairs to the washing machine and call that an exercise program? This is a question the experts on the panel wrestled with as well. Can you accumulate exercise piecemeal—say, in several bouts of activity as short as a few minutes during the course of a normal, busy day?

The most direct evidence that piecemeal exercise "counts" toward improving your health comes from studies like the one by Robert DeBusk at Stanford, which compared men who did three 10- minute bouts of moderate to vigorous activity a day with men who worked out for one continuous 30-minute period. Cardiorespiratory fitness improved significantly in both groups. But since the exercise in this and most similar studies is fairly intense, the results don't necessarily apply to more moderate activities like housework. They do, however, support the idea that the total amount of exercise matters more than doing it all in one session, and the exercise patterns in epidemiological studies like MRFIT back this up.

In addition, Rena Wing's group has found that encouraging people to do multiple short bouts of exercise leads to more total exercise per day than telling them to slog through one long workout. That result shoots right to heart of the sedentary psyche. When it comes to increasing physical activity, for most people getting motivated to start is generally the hardest part. Wing's research suggests that people may have an easier time starting a workout when they know their pain will be short-lived.

If squeezing exercise in a few minutes here and there is what works best with your schedule, it's going to improve your health. That seems to be the most reasonable message to take away from the research. A short workout is certainly better than nothing at all, and it may even be as beneficial as that half-hour aerobics class. Then again, if you can't manage even this much exercise, a drove of pharmaceutical companies is now working to give you the same kind of metabolic lift without ever leaving the confines of your Barcalounger.

FIVE

The Armchair Workout

WILL THERE EVER BE A PILL THAT WILL MAKE US THIN?

In December 1994, Pam Ruff, a cardiac sonographer at the MeritCare Medical Center in Fargo, North Dakota, noticed something unusual in the medical files of two female patients. Echocardiograms of the relatively young women's hearts showed that they both suffered from a condition that is rare in people under the age of 50: leaky valves. The tiny doors that close off the chambers in their hearts weren't sealing properly, and some of the blood was trickling back through them. As a result, their hearts were working harder to keep blood flowing. When Ruff looked at the women's files, she discovered that the two young women also had something else in common. They had both taken a popular combination of diet drugs known as fen-phen.

This weight-loss treatment had grown in popularity ever since a 1992 clinical trial by pharmacologist Michael Weintraub, then at the University of Rochester in New

York. Weintraub combined the appetite suppressant fen-fluramine and the nonaddictive amphetemine-like drug phentermine in an effort to help obese people lose weight. Fenfluramine boosts serotonin, a brain chemical respon-sible for feelings of satiety and well-being. Phentermine increases the levels of norepinephrine and dopamine in the brain, causing people to eat faster but stop eating sooner. Neither drug on its own had been particularly effective in helping people lose weight. But Weintraub showed that by using half doses of each of them, people could get better long-term weight-loss results than with either drug alone.

Since both fenfluramine and phentermine had been on the market for over two decades with no reports of valve trouble, Weintraub never expected safety to be an issue. Nor did Ruff's colleagues at MeritCare, who assumed that the link between the heart problems and the diet drugs was a coincidence. But Ruff was unwilling to shrug it off. Over the next two years, she collected files on about 20 fen-phen users—all with similar, rare valve disorders—who passed through the MeritCare cardiography lab.

Then in December 1996, MeritCare cardiologist Jack Crary saw a patient who had a valve problem that clearly had not been there several months earlier, before the woman had started taking fen-phen. As Crary spoke to this patient, the suspicions that Ruff had voiced suddenly crystallized in his mind. He looked back at the cases she had collected and found that they made a convincing case for a link. Crary then contacted cardiologists at the Mayo Clinic in Rochester, Minnesota, and found that they too had noticed an unusual valve disorder a year earlier in a woman who had been taking fen-phen. They had since seen other diet drug users with the same problem.

Together the doctors from the two medical centers compiled 24 cases of fen-phen users who had leaky heart valves. They wrote up their findings for the August 28, 1997, issue of the *New England Journal of Medicine*. Because the health threat these findings implied was so great, the journal allowed the doctors to announce their results in a press conference on July 8. At that time, the Food and Drug Administration asked doctors nationwide to report any other associations between the diet drugs and heart problems. By the end of August the agency had amassed 101 cases.

In some of these cases, the patients took fenfluramine without phentermine, or they used a drug that had only recently entered the market: Redux. Redux is dexfenfluramine, a chemical form of fenfluramine that the body is able to process with fewer side effects. It gained FDA approval in April 1996, and use of it immediately soared, both as a stand-alone treatment and as a substitute for the fenfluramine in fen-phen. Redux was averaging 80,000 prescriptions a week when the reports of valve damage began to appear.

By then the number of people taking one of the fenfluramine drugs was so large that doctors from five medical centers around the United States had no difficulty responding to an additional request by the FDA. The physicians were asked to look for heart problems in people who had taken either Redux or fenfluramine with no cardiac complaint. Out of 291 patients, nearly a third turned out to have valve damage that had previously gone undetected. Based on this evidence, the FDA asked the manufacturers of Redux and fenfluramine to pull them off the market on September 15, 1997. The agency also advised anyone who had taken these drugs to seek medical attention.

The events marked an abrupt end to America's whirlwind romance with these diet drugs. Yet in many ways they merely served as an introduction to a much broader story: the emergence of a new generation of weight-loss pills. Two months after Redux and fenfluramine went off the market, the FDA granted approval to another diet drug: Meridia. Known clinically as sibutramine, Meridia is product of the Knoll Pharmaceutical Company. It is an appetite suppressant that slows dissipation of the brain chemicals norepinephrine and, to a lesser extent, serotonin. In contrast to Redux and fenfluramine, Meridia does not stimulate the release of serotonin—only its reabsorption at the nerve endings. Nevertheless, its effect on that brain chemical, and the worries this raised, prompted FDA officials to announce that they had found no evidence that Meridia poses the same risk of heart valve damage as the recalled drugs. As for its effectiveness, Meridia is comparable to its predecessors. In clinical trials, it produced weight losses that were seven to eleven pounds better than placebo after a year, or about 15 pounds overall.

Close on Meridia's heels in the FDA approval process is Xenical from Hoffman-LaRoche. Clinically known as orlistat, it is the first of an entirely new class of diet drugs.

Instead of acting on brain chemistry, Xenical interferes with an intestinal enzyme that breaks down dietary fat. In doing so it prevents about 30 percent of the fat people eat from being absorbed by their bodies. Combined with a program of diet, exercise, and behavior therapy, its effects on weight are comparable to those of Meridia. Obese patients lose an average of eight pounds more than people taking placebo. They also see improvements in their cholesterol, blood pressure, and blood sugar levels.

While Meridia and Xenical are likely to be the last drugs approved by the FDA before the year 2000, research on weight-control medications is moving forward at a rapid pace. By one recent count, 62 new compounds for treating obesity are in various stages of testing and development. "I expect we'll see one or two new drugs being submitted to us every year for the next five to ten years," says Leo Lutwak, a medical officer with the FDA's Center for Drug Evaluation and Research. Redux and fen-phen, the first diet drugs to stake their claim to the brave new world of the dieting future, were only the first trickle of a tidal wave of diet drugs to come.

Depending on your aversion to the idea of putting chemicals in your body, this deluge of new weight-loss aids sounds like either a great idea or a horrible one. But really, tinkering with weight on this biomolecular level is no different from what doctors have been doing for decades to treat other ailments like ulcers, manic depression or hypertension. The difference is that historically, physicians haven't seen obesity as occupying the same camp as these other chronic conditions.

That view has changed dramatically over the last few years, in part because of the failure of traditional methods of diet, exercise, and behavioral therapy. Doctors who treated obese patients using these accepted methods simply grew frustrated. But an even greater driving force has been research on the genetic roots of obesity and on the chemical signals that strictly regulate eating. These lie at the root of a growing sense among weight specialists that obesity isn't a simple product of overeating or lack of willpower. The problem is largely biological.

During the late 1980s obesity researchers, particularly those in the North American Association for the Study of Obesity (NAASO), began to refer to obesity as a disease— a chronic condition that requires chronic treatment. More and more, they expressed dissatisfaction with the medications available to treat this condition. What was needed, they felt, was an array of drugs that could help people in the lifelong struggle to maintain healthy weights.

To that end, NAASO leaders began a quiet campaign to convince the Food and Drug Administration that such drugs had to be held to a different standard than diet drugs of the past. Weight-loss aids have, for decades, been considered ineffective if the weight lost while people were taking the drugs came right back after they stopped. But this thinking didn't make much sense if obesity was truly a chronic condition like hypertension. If a doctor put you on an ACE inhibitor to treat your blood pressure and it worked, he or she wouldn't immediately take you off the drug and expect the effect to persist. Nor would the doctor attribute the rebound of your blood pressure to lack of willpower. Yet that was the logic applied to diet drugs both by the FDA and by medical professionals.

In their writings and their conversations with FDA officials, NAASO members repeatedly pointed out this double standard. In 1994, largely as a result of these efforts, the FDA issued a new set of guidelines for the evaluation of drugs for obesity. Where drug companies once saw only resistance to diet drugs from the regulatory agency, they now saw a green light. That change and the quickening pace of molecular research moved antiobesity medications to the top of the drug companies' agendas.

The Next Generation of Diet Drugs

The fact that the tools of modern molecular biology are finally being applied to the study of weight is one reason to believe that the diet drugs now in development won't be as clumsy and ineffective as those we have seen in the past. Obesity is now an area of study as legitimate as heart disease or cancer therapy. As scientists have accrued inklings of how the body's weight-control machinery works, they have quickly mined those insights for new treatment strategies.

No one knew before 1994, for example, about the leptin protein. Since then, it has jump started the entire field of obesity research by revealing the connections within connections of the body's weight-control apparatus and by providing scientists with new insights into which targets to aim for with their drugs. Leptin itself is being tested as a drug, naturally. In contrast to the hopes raised when it was first discovered, however, few believe that it is going to have the same kind of immediate and immense "skinnying" effect on people the way it did on the *ob* mouse.

In general, people don't become obese because they don't have enough leptin in their bloodstreams, as was the case with the *ob* mouse. In fact people who are overweight generally overproduce leptin. Their bodies seem to have developed a resistance to it, or at least that is the assumption that has been made because of the similarity to the way people with type II diabetes manage to produce insulin but for some reason are resistant to its effects. Type II diabetes can, however, be treated effectively with additional insulin.

Experiments in mice support the idea that giving overweight people more leptin may also have an effect. Leptin causes weight loss in DIO mice—the rodents that seem to be most like the majority of overweight people because they gain weight when fed a high-fat diet. For that reason, no one has ruled out the possibility that leptin therapy may decrease appetite and lead to weight loss in many obese people. Like the insulin treatment, this sort of therapy may not be a solution to someone's weight problem, but it could be an effective stopgap measure.

Amgen, a California-based biotechnology company, has pinned a good deal of hope on this possibility. They paid Rockefeller University $20 million for an exclusive license to develop products based on the leptin gene. In May 1996, Amgen began the first human clinical trials of leptin. Such "phase 1" trials are mainly designed to test the safety of a drug and how well people tolerate different doses, but they also give strong hints about how effective a drug will be.

In June 1997, Amgen reported that 30 to 45 percent of the people who completed 28 days of the trial with optimal doses of leptin lost at least 4 pounds. For comparison, 19 percent of the people who received a placebo lost that much. People who stayed in the study even longer, 90 days instead of 28, lost 4 to 9 pounds compared with only 3 pounds for those on placebo. These results were positive enough to prompt Amgen to move on to phase 2 trials, which are geared more toward establishing leptin's effectiveness in treating obesity. As it turned out, phase 2 showed that leptin was no more effective than a placebo in helping a group of obese people lose weight. But within this group was a subset of people for whom leptin was effective. And Amgen claims that they can identify, before treatment, who will respond to leptin and who won't.

Throughout this testing period, Amgen has also been developing two leptin-like molecules, known in the industry as mimetics. The reason for this, according to Amgen's spokesperson, was "to address the possible lack of patient acceptance of leptin at higher doses." The main side effects seen in the phase one trials were injection-site reactions from these higher doses. Trial subjects receiving as many as three shots of leptin a day developed skin irritations from the injections. "That says to me that they were trying to put tons of this material into these people," says Margaret Van Heek, a drug developer at Schering-Plough. That Amgen is going forward with a mimetic that can be tolerated at higher doses implies that people will need massive amounts of the drug to show an effect.

What's more, even large doses of leptin may not work for everyone. A study by Andrew Greenberg, who directs obesity research at Tufts University and at the New England Medical Center in Boston, found that out of the eight people in the phase one trial who received the highest drug dose, one lost no weight at all. Another gained weight.

A more fruitful treatment strategy may be to determine why some people aren't responding to the already high levels of leptin in their bloodstreams. One of the researchers involved in this strategy is L. Arthur Campfield, who directs the leptin project at Hoffmann-LaRoche in Nutley, New Jersey. As one who has struggled with weight himself, Campfield is passionate about finding the biological roots of eating, particularly in the brain. "There's this whole series of signals that are integrated by a neural network in the brain," he says. "And these neurons make decisions like when you'll start to eat, and for how long you will eat, and when you will stop eating."

Leptin and its receptors (there are several different receptors in different regions of the brain) are a key part of this network. By looking at the ways leptin interacts with other parts of the system, researchers are beginning to see how the many pieces fit together. Leptin is known, for example, to decrease the levels of the brain chemical neuropeptide Y (NPY), the powerful booster of appetite. Leptin also works its magic on a series of compounds and receptors in the brain called the melanocortin system.

This system is another one of the body's routes for controlling food intake and body weight.

Using these and other examples, Campfield has theorized that leptin may play the role of "conductor" to all these disparate elements of the weight-regulating system. Like Keith Lockhart, who leads the Boston Pops, it may bring up the volume on the satiety signals when it is in large supply and at the same time tone down the brain chemicals like NPY that make us hungry. For now, the details of this weight-control orchestra are still sketchy. But as researchers begin to understand it on a molecular level, Campfield says, pharmaceutical companies like his "will bring everything we have to bear on developing drugs so that people can start eating less often, eat less at each meal, store less body fat, have a lower body weight and have improved health."

Burn This

To that list, Campfield also adds expending more energy, which would be across the orchestra pit from the section that controls appetite. A host of brain chemicals continuously control how much energy we burn, not only when we exercise but in our day to day activities of waking, eating, and lounging around the house. Drug companies are equally driven to exploit this side of the weight-control apparatus.

One of their favorite targets has been the beta-3 receptor, a biochemical switch that can turn fat cells into fat-burning engines. Beta-3 receptors lie on the surface of a particular type of fat called brown fat. Unlike white fat cells, which store energy by storing fat molecules, brown fat cells burn fat and dissipate the energy as heat. A compound that could attach to beta-3 receptors and turn on the brown fat engine could be an ideal weight-loss drug. Researchers say that it would provide many of the benefits of regular mild exercise.

A handful of drug companies would have had such an "exercise pill" on the market long before now had they not encountered a few potholes along the way. During the late 1980s, scientists from Hoffman-La Roche and the British-based companies SmithKline Beecham and ICI (now Zeneca) tested a few carefully selected compounds in people for the first time and found that these drugs just didn't work the way they did in laboratory animals.

For the scientists to see any measurable effect on metabolism, the drugs had to be given in such high doses that they had serious side effects. They caused the recipients' hands to shake, sometimes severely, prompting a few subjects to withdraw from the trials. The drugs also boosted heart rate. They produced very little heat and hardly any weight loss. The side effects far outweighed the drug's benefits, and the researchers brought the clinical trials to an end.

But the efforts weren't a total waste. The trials made it clear to researchers just exactly why the drugs were causing these side effects in people. The problem was that the compounds were great at locking onto beta-3 receptors in rats, but the human version of this molecule had a slightly different shape. Which meant that at high doses, the drugs were swimming around patients' bodies, occasionally hooking up with beta-3 receptors but also acting on a variety of other related receptors and generally leaving havoc in their wake.

All the drug companies needed to eliminate the nasty side effects was a compound that would stick to the human beta-3 receptor exclusively. The cloning of that receptor in 1993 put the beta-3 drug program back on track. It allowed the drug companies to screen thousands of substances from their armamentaria for those that tightly embrace the human receptor. Since then, Merck, SmithKline Beecham, Squibb, Pfizer, and Eli Lilly have all filed patent applications for compounds that selectively target the human beta-3 receptor. Clinical trials of the compounds have begun, and though company executives aren't divulging any secrets, they are smiling. Jamie Dananberg, who arrived at Eli Lilly in 1996 to direct their clinical development program for beta-3 drugs, pronounces himself "really pleased with our development. That's what I can tell you."

The companies still have to clear a couple of scientific hurdles, though. One is that researchers have never been able to find a great deal of brown fat in fully grown people. In most animals, at any stage of life, brown fat is gathered in clearly defined pads, like a separate organ system. It lies near the kidneys, near the heart, and underneath the shoulder blades. Oddly enough, in humans the same is true only of infants. Brown fat seems to function only in the first few weeks of a newborn's life.

Jean Himms-Hagen, a biochemist at the University of Ottawa in Ontario and a renowned authority on brown fat, has long studied this puzzle. One day when she was holding her newborn grandson, shortly after he had eaten, she noticed how warm he was. That gave her the idea that the heat produced by brown fat cells might be used to tell babies when to cry out for food and when to stop eating. She later attached a thermometer to her grandchild, as well as to a handful of other newborns, and showed that the temperature does indeed rise steadily from a minimum when the child cries out to be fed to a maximum when, sated, he or she pulls away from the mother's breast.

Until the child learns to respond to other cues of hunger and satiety, the brown fat seems to be providing a signal. But as the child begins to develop, its brown fat cells gradually fade from the picture. In adults the fat pads are dispersed. Researchers now know that the cells still exist; they are merely in the background, blending in with other cells around the major organs and blood vessels. They're also empty of fat molecules. But this little hitch hasn't stopped the search for beta-3 drugs; the companies involved are willing to gamble that beta-3 compounds are going to turn human brown fat cells, wherever they may be, into active, fat-stoked furnaces.

The desire of drug companies to hedge their bets, however, has led to a surge of interest in another family of molecules called the uncoupling proteins (UCPs). These are the proteins inside the brown fat that allow it to dissipate energy. UCP literally "uncouples" the engine that usually turns fat into a chemical form of saved energy and allows the brown cell to churn out heat instead.

When this protein was first identified in the mid-1970s, it wasn't immediately targeted as an antiobesity drug because of the belief that brown fat was active only in babies. In recent years, researchers have discovered a host of other uncoupling proteins—four so far, and there may be more—in tissues throughout the body. The original UCP is only in brown fat. UCP2, cloned in March 1997, turns out to be in white fat cells as well as other tissues. UCP3, which showed up later the same year, is in both brown fat and muscle in laboratory animals but only in muscle in humans. UCP4 has not yet been cloned, but a UCP has been found in potatoes, which produce it when they're exposed to cold.

This emerging family of proteins has stirred up enormous excitement within the drug-development community, because where researchers once thought that only brown fat could dissipate energy, they now believe that a wide variety of cells have this capacity. Drug developers are particularly interested in UCP2 because this protein is in white fat cells, and if there's one thing people have a lot of in their bodies, it is white fat.

"The fact that it's in white adipocytes is important," says Duke University obesity researcher Richard Surwit, "because the real question is going to be, Can you turn on uncoupling proteins in specific organs? You don't want to turn them on, for instance, in the heart. And I'm not sure you'd want to turn them on in muscle, because what uncoupling does is divert energy from the creation of ATP, which is the source of energy for all biologic functions. . . . So if you were to do this in muscle, then you could predict that a person who had highly activated uncoupling activity in muscle would have muscle atrophy. They wouldn't be making muscle tissue." But fat atrophy would be okay with almost everybody. If researchers could figure out a way to switch on the uncoupling protein in white fat, that would truly be a weight loss drug with substantial impact.

Researchers and drug developers are also excited about UCP2 because it is affected by diet. Not only is UCP2 in white fat, it is turned on by a high-fat diet—at least in certain obesity-resistant animals. The animals that have the ability to turn on UCP2 when they eat a lot of fat can obviously burn the fat very quickly, which is why Surwit thinks UCP2 may be a key to why some people can eat all the fatty foods they want and not gain weight.

One more interesting thing about this protein: in laboratory animals, UCP2 mirrors whatever leptin is doing in the bloodstream. Levels of both compounds either go up in response to fatty foods or not, depending on whether the animals are resistant or susceptible to obesity. Leptin once again seems to be at the center of things—between fatty foods, in this case, and efficient fat burning in animals, and possibly people, who are naturally resistant to weight gain.

Such stories of connections upon connections keep popping up now that researchers are using leptin to tie together different aspects of weight regulation. The examples discussed here are only a hint of the fascinating loops that molecular biologist have uncovered since they began applying their tools to the problem of weight control. They give rise to the feeling that researchers are finally beginning to understand just how the body regulates weight.

Novel drugs that emerge from this newfound understanding will target various aspects of the body's weight control system. They should, therefore, be more specific and more effective than the diet drugs we have seen so far. That is particularly true in the case of Redux and fen-phen. The new way of thinking about obesity may have eased Redux's journey through the FDA, but both of the fenfluramine drugs came out of research that dated back three decades.

The problems encountered with these drugs are nonetheless closely entwined with our skewed attitude toward fat. And that is a snake that is likely to bite again, as more and more weight-loss drugs come onto the market. If we approach these new drugs in the same way we approached Redux and fen-phen, we're likely to have similar disasters on our hands. To get to the promised land of effective weight-loss drugs, we will all have to become a lot more savvy about how we put them to use.

Redux Redux

In a culture where you can scarcely find a women's magazine without the words "thin" or "thighs" on the cover, it's no surprise that Redux and fen-phen fell into the hands of people of all weights. A "get 'em while they're hot" mentality prevailed. Federal health officials estimate that between 1.2 and 4.7 million Americans used these drugs before they were pulled off pharmacists' shelves.

This was in spite of the fact that the drugs were approved only for the treatment of people who were clinically obese. What's more, in 1996 a group comprising some of the country's most eminent obesity researchers and clinicians recommended against the routine use of diet drugs to treat even obese individuals. The National Task Force on the Prevention and Treatment of Obesity (NTFPTO) said that the benefits and costs of long-term drug treatment outweighed the risks only for those people who were obese and suffering from related health conditions, such as diabetes or high blood pressure.

The task force was, of course, referring to the known risks at the time. The heart valve problem didn't show up until 1997. But Redux and fenfluramine were known to increase the risk of primary pulmonary hypertension, or PPH, by 23 to 46 times. PPH is a condition in which the blood vessels to the lungs constrict, putting undue pressure on the heart's walls. Since only about one person in a million ordinarily develops PPH, the risk from the diet drugs was still relatively small. But PPH is a progressive disease for which there is no cure. Approximately half of the people who get PPH die within four years. Anyone taking these diet drugs, even if they were obese and suffering from related conditions, should have been advised to carefully consider the risks alongside the potential benefits.

If they weren't obese—well, it's hard to believe that millions of people with only mild weight problems would have flocked to Redux and fen-phen if they had actually understood what these drugs were supposed to do. The reality of these diet pills was that they were intended for use with a serious program of diet, exercise and behavior modification. That's because they weren't simple fat melters. What they did was work on the system that regulates appetite. They also reduced the body's set-point, or the weight it defends, which made cutting back on food a little easier. But without the other weight-loss measures, the drugs had trivial effects.

While taking a prescribed course of these drugs, people lost, on average, about 10 percent of their starting weight. Most of the weight loss took place during the first six months of treatment and then more or less stabilized as long as the people stayed on the medications. If they went off, the weight came back because the drugs were no longer decreasing the body's set-point. This meant that people had to stay on the diet drugs potentially for the rest of their lives in order to lose just 10 percent of their weight.

The drugs of the future, while they may be more effective than the ones we have seen so far, are likely to have many of the same characteristics. They will be intended for people who are clinically obese; they will be used in long-term treatments; and they will be geared toward use with a program of diet and exercise. More specifically, such a program will be a requirement for FDA approval of any new drug as far as any of the interested parties dare to see into the future.

A handful of obesity researchers, like George Bray at the Pennington Biomedical Research Center in Baton Rouge, don't believe these other measures will be necessary once effective drugs are developed. But the vast majority say that there will never be a pill that will let you eat what you want, remain sedentary, and not gain weight.

What they hope is that drugs will make it possible for people whose obesity is a serious health risk to maintain a diet and exercise program and lose weight with much less struggle.

The diet drugs of the future will also have side effects. Examples of this are already apparent for both Meridia and Xenical. Meridia induces large, potentially dangerous increases in blood pressure in a subset of patients who take it. For most people the blood pressure rise is just two to three points (millimeters of mercury). This is a negligible increase. But 4 to 10 percent of patients who used the drug in clinical trials had blood pressure rises of 10 to 15 points. Such an increase could lead to a heart attack, stroke, or other life-threatening ailments.

Based largely on these increases and the lack of information about them, the FDA's own panel of scientific advisors, who met on September 26, 1996, to consider Meridia's approval, voted five to four that the benefits of the drug did not outweigh its risks. After that meeting, Knoll officials convinced the FDA that it would be possible to know, soon after a patient started taking the drug, whether he or she was a candidate for such side effects. Within their existing database, Knoll had evidence that most of the increases in either systolic or diastolic blood pressure occurred within the first four weeks of treatment. FDA officials were satisfied that if doctors monitored a patient's blood pressure diligently, they would be able to identify any aberrations early and immediately take the patient off the drug to halt its effects. After the drug was approved, consumer advocates went one step further, advising consumers to monitor their own blood pressure for added safety.

As for Xenical, there are obvious drawbacks to a drug that dumps fat into a person's stools. For the same reasons that olestra's warning label on gastric disturbances and anal leakage has fueled legions of jokes, Xenical's side effects of diarrhea, loose stools and foul odor are likely to turn off a few potential users. These are not life threatening, but they are the kinds of things that might drive your friends to do an intervention. Curtis Jatkauskas, a Colorado resident who signed on as a guinea pig for one of the early clinical trials of Xenical, said he knew after a few days that he was on the drug, not the placebo, because "it was just like taking a bottle of oil and throwing it in the toilet." His odd, but perhaps prophetic, reaction to this knowledge was to go ahead and eat all the cheeseburgers he wanted.

An even more disturbing problem that stalled Xenical's widely anticipated 1997 FDA approval is an increased incidence of breast cancer in patients taking the drug in clinical studies. During their review of the drug, FDA scientists noticed that the number of cases of breast cancer in the clinical trials was unusually high. One out of every 68 women taking the optimal dose of 120 milligrams of Xenical three times a day received a diagnosis of breast cancer compared to only one out of 316 women taking a smaller dose and one out of 234 taking placebo.

During a meeting of the FDA's scientific advisory committee on March 13, 1998, scientists from Hoffman-LaRoche presented evidence that Xenical did not cause or promote the tumor growth and that the cancer cases could reasonably be attributed to chance. Bruce Stadel, a Medical Officer at the FDA who analyzed the breast cancer data, considered chance to be within the realm of possibility, but was markedly concerned about evidence implying that something was causing tumors to grow while people were on the drug. The FDA's panel of scientific advisors deadlocked five to five over whether the overall benefits of Xenical outweighed its risks.

Such risks, as well as the lesser side effects of weight-loss medications, will loom even larger in the years to come because doctors will be more likely to prescribe several diet drugs simultaneously. Based on early experiences with Redux and fen-phen, it is becoming increasingly clear that the body cannot be easily tricked into giving up the fat stores it holds so dear. One of the most widely recognized examples of this tenacity is that these diet drugs, when they were taken individually, had a 10-percent ceiling on how much weight loss they produced. That may be because these first-generation drugs were weak. But to many researchers, that consistent plateau implies that there may be biological constraints on how much a drug can do before the body starts defending itself vigorously.

Further evidence of those constraints comes from the fact that in the few truly long-term studies that exist, people on appetite suppressants have seen their weight start to rebound after three years, even though they continue to take the drugs. Richard Atkinson, a University of Wisconsin obesity researcher who ran one such study, says that his impression was that people were less motivated over time.

The excitement of the initial weight loss had worn off. The memory of what it was like to be 30 or 40 pounds heavier faded. And the incentive to keep up a sensible diet and exercise program waned. But Atkinson readily admits that nobody really knows why this rebound occurs.

The rebound as well as the 10-percent ceiling raise the question of whether it's possible to design a weight-loss drug that tweaks the system in a specific way without the body compensating for that change. "Twenty-odd years ago we thought we could manipulate body weight by increasing metabolism or by appetite suppression," says one independent drug consultant. "But I think now everybody agrees this is a very closed loop. Maybe one closed loop, maybe several." Weight, metabolism, and appetite are all tightly coupled within the body.

"Food intake is so primary, so central to survival, that it makes sense that there are going to be fail-safe mechanisms telling an organism, 'Hey, I'm hungry, I need to eat,'" says Xavier Pi-Sunyer, director of the Obesity Research Center at Columbia University College of Physicians and Surgeons. "So you block one path and another path takes its place." For these reasons, many researchers believe that in order to successfully treat obesity, patients may have to take a cocktail of drugs that target different aspects of the weight-control system. One may dampen appetite while another boosts metabolism. A third could work on the body's ability to absorb fat.

The idea that combination therapy is the way to go has already become so firmly entrenched that even before the fenfluramines were taken off the market, diet doctors and weight-loss centers began advertising a host of other drug duos based on scant scientific reasoning. One popular treatment has been phen-Pro, which replaces fenfluramine with Prozac, another serotonin-boosting drug, even though weight loss on Prozac alone has been shown to be minimal and short-lived. Diet doctors are also prescribing phen-chrom, which includes the mineral supplement chromium picolinate. Despite this compound's reputation as a weight-loss wonder drug, the Federal Trade Commission has recently cracked down on companies who make that claim, citing the lack of scientific evidence. On the contrary, studies have suggested that chromium picolinate supplements may increase the risk of some cancers.

The "natural" alternative to these drug concoctions has been herbal fen-phen. This is a mix of ephedra, a natural stimulant, and other herbs. Combinations of ephedra and caffeine have been studied in clinical trials and shown to be mildly effective for treatment of obesity. But while ephedra is derived from the Chinese herb *ma huang* and has been used for centuries, it can be as potent and dangerous as any drug even when taken in the recommended dosage. Ephedra has been linked to more than 15 deaths nationwide and hundreds of adverse events including strokes and seizures. Such examples make it clear that with multiple drug therapies, the potential for cross reactions and compounding side effects is even greater. This and the other characteristics of the diet drugs to come make thoughtful prescription of these medications by doctors more crucial than ever.

The Good Doctor

In the world in which obesity is being redefined as a medical condition, it is unfortunate that experience with fen-phen and Redux has shown doctors to be culpable. It was they after all, who wrote millions of prescriptions for these diet drugs, often for purely cosmetic purposes. Some doctors were simply lured by the quick buck. From Boston to Los Angeles, signs were posted on telephone poles advertising 30 pounds of weight loss in 30 days for 30 bucks. Those doing the offering were little more than black market vendors for diet pills. Patients who took the bait often had only cursory contact with a physician. They were given lists of possible side effects and told to monitor themselves for any reactions.

Perhaps people who chose to play a game of chance with their health by responding to such ads had only themselves to blame. But even people who managed to steer clear of quacks and hucksters often found themselves in the hands of doctors who misunderstood what these drugs were about. Bernard McNamara, director of Weight Control Medical Associates in Burbank, California, had some of his patients on a weight-maintenance program in which he told them that they didn't have to take the diet drugs he prescribed every day, but only on those occasions when they felt they needed "a little help to resist cravings." That, says obesity specialist Richard Atkinson, "is absolutely insane—like saying if you've got diabetes, when you feel bad take a little insulin."

It hasn't really sunk in that today's diet drugs are long-term medications. Both doctors and patients are still thinking of them as quick-fix solutions instead of an accompaniment to lifelong changes in diet, activity, and eating behaviors. This is partly a leftover from the 1960s and 1970s, when the diet drugs in use were amphetamines that led to severe problems with addiction and abuse. These drugs were approved only for short-term use to keep people from becoming dependent on them.

Now, even though addiction is no longer a factor, it's still hard for us to adjust to the concept that diet drugs, like most medications, are effective only as long as they are used. The notion of getting thin and then quitting the drugs simply no longer applies. In misunderstanding what the drugs can do and misrepresenting them to patients, doctors are merely repeating the mistakes of the past. They are taking the scientific understanding of obesity treatment and applying it so wrongly that it might as well be snake oil.

It is impossible to escape the fact that doctors grow up in the same fat-phobic culture as everyone else. The culture profoundly influences the idea that obesity is a disease that can be treated with drugs, often transforming it into the belief that obesity is a condition to be fought at all costs. Many doctors still find it easier to believe that fat is the enemy than to diagnose and treat the underlying problems. This bias undermines the only real goal: health.

Healthy people come in a variety of shapes and sizes. Even if all the biochemical idiosyncrasies about how our bodies regulate weight are "fixed" by some pill or combination of pills, the vast majority of us would still not look like the people we see on television. *Baywatch* bodies are, at best, an anomaly of nature; in fact, on some, nature's hand had less influence than that of a good plastic surgeon. Only by accepting a little bit of what nature delivers in its wide spectrum of human shapes and sizes will doctors and patients be able to make rational choices.

With this in mind, thoughtful researchers have begun to advocate an alternative approach to obesity treatment. "There's a consensus within the research community," says Hoffmann-LaRoche's Art Campfield, "and it's starting to get now into the patient community, that it's not how much you weigh or how much body fat you have that should be the focus of treatment, or even the thing by which we measure success for dieting and exercise. Instead it's how healthy you are. So what we've coined is a term called metabolic fitness. The idea is, if you have an obese person who is hypertensive and has elevated triglycerides, what you'd like to do is help them lose enough weight so that those things go back into the normal range. And that's good enough. They don't have to look like Cindy Crawford."

Metabolic fitness rather than the pursuit of thinness—Michael Weintraub learned this lesson during the original fen-phen trial. In a summary of his results, Weintraub wrote that he and his colleagues had "erred seriously" in attempting to bring patients to a predetermined weight rather than measuring success by the fact that people could maintain a weight loss or keep from gaining weight over the course of the four-year study. Their bias was understandable. Most dieters strive toward the goal of an ideal weight. Yet with such an outlook, Weintraub wrote, "failure will be inevitable, the regain of lost weight will be highly likely, and the potential for a 'roller coaster' or 'yo-yo' situation will be created." Only by embracing such lessons will doctors and patients get to the point where these drugs might live up to their potential.

Better Living Through Chemistry

Perhaps the most ardent believer in the potential of antiobesity drugs is George Bray, director of the Pennington Biomedical Research Center in Baton Rouge, Louisiana. Pennington lies just past a cluster of fast-food restaurants scattered along a four-lane highway. A broad, low fountain splashes through a dozen configurations on the Center's vast manicured grounds.

Inside, the atmosphere is plush. A gold-framed portrait of Bray hangs just outside his second-floor office. Bray stands with one foot resting on a curb, looking athletic and wiry. He has spent a 40-year career telling people to diet and exercise in order to lose weight, yet he has come to the conclusion that these are not the solutions to America's rising tide of obesity.

Is that because diets and exercise don't work? "Oh, if you do it seriously enough they help a lot," Bray says. "But we aren't going to be that serious. You know, if you ran five miles every day and ate a low fat diet, then everybody would be thin, or almost. It's very clear that you can keep weight down for years if you make some regular and continued changes in your behavior. But we're not going to get people to do that. . . . We all sit behind the wheel of our cars and we park as close to where we work as we can and we sit in nice air-conditioned offices and we don't get out and exercise very much. Some people do. I mean there are people jogging around Boston Common, the Mall in Washington, Central Park. But those are usually thin people to start with."

What Bray believes in are drugs. He thinks that as researchers develop increasingly effective drugs for obesity, the need for diets and exercise will go way down. "If you've got good drugs the drugs work," he says. "It isn't dieting when you're not wanting to eat. I've been this weight for 45 years and I'm not deprived. Something in my system says this is sufficient, and whatever will happen with drugs will be the same thing."

To arguments that diet drugs are being misused and misprescribed, Bray, like many obesity researchers, says this is a problem of physician education, not an indictment of the drugs. Bray has even gone so far as to write that the abuse of weight loss drugs by people who only want to lose 10 or 20 pounds is "a price that may be justifiable" in order to have drugs to reduce the risk of death from diabetes, hypertension, and heart disease in people who are truly obese.

He likens the current situation with obesity drugs to the days of blood pressure treatment before the first antihypertensive medications came out in the late 1950s. "People were using very low-sodium diet," he says, "and you could lower peoples' blood pressure with very low-sodium diet. But as soon as the good pharmacologic agents came along, almost all the attention to the other approaches waned."

The same thing happened with anticholesterol medications during the 1980s. "The cholesterol education program says do all these great dietary things and then if your cholesterol is still where it was you can take drugs," says Bray. "Well, for practical purposes everybody's getting their statin drugs very early on because it's so much more effective. And most people aren't prepared to eat 50 grams of fiber every day with a zero cholesterol diet and no saturated fat. People aren't prepared to do that."

Whether or not you agree with Bray's assessment of what people are capable of doing, he is strikingly honest about his reasoning. In his no-nonsense way, Bray articulates the thoughts of many of his colleagues and the frustrations that have driven them towards pharmaceutical solutions. They have tried other approaches and found them lacking. The weight-control system they are fighting is too tenacious. The high-fat, sedentary culture in which they are doing battle has too many Americans in its grip. The diet drugs now in development take the war on fat to a molecular level. In the past few years, researchers have seen just enough of the weight-control system to be convinced that these medications are the best hope for an end to the epidemic of obesity.

SIX

Facing Fat

THE STRUGGLE FOR
SIZE ACCEPTANCE

It is late afternoon in the ballroom of a downtown New Orleans hotel, 80 miles from George Bray's office and a world away in terms of attitude. Marilyn Wann, a vivacious woman who goes by the nickname Hank, is sashaying down a runway clad in a snappy black-and-white beach wrap. A driving rock beat amplifies the sway of her hips. She glides to a stop in front of a British Broadcasting (BBC) camera crew perched at the end of the catwalk and strikes her best supermodel pose. An appreciative whoop rises from the audience. It isn't every day a girl gets to play fashion model, and Wann has the room in the palm of her hand.

Overnight her hair has gone from punk, bottle white to a shocking shade of pink, which perfectly matches a lacy little number she will change into for the lingerie section of the fashion show. That lingerie is being modeled at all on this day is an act of revolutionary defiance, for

Wann and all the other models in the show are fat. And today they are letting it all hang out, in loose flowing clothing draped over their large, undulating bodies—not camouflaging black, but reds and florals and clingy cloth. There is cleavage to die for and nary a cinched waist in sight.

This flouting of the usual fashion ethic is one of the highlights of a week-long convention of NAAFA, the National Association to Advance Fat Acceptance. Founded in 1969 as a nonprofit organization offering advocacy and support for fat people, NAAFA has since grown to about 5,000 members. It is one of the oldest participants in a small but vocal size-acceptance movement that is challenging the redefinition of obesity as a disease and working to turn our media-driven aversion to fat on its head.

There's no getting away from it; seeing fat people all around absolutely shifts your world view. Just a couple of hours among the NAAFA folks at this annual convention makes everyone else look intensely skinny. Even the merely overweight people in the ballroom, after a while, look a little too light to really belong to this group. This is exactly the effect that NAAFA is aiming for: an environment where fat people feel not only welcome, but often, for the first time in their lives, normal. The members attending this annual meeting can move through the activities of life without fear of harassment. And the operative word here is move. Rather than letting their shame at being fat keep them closeted and sedentary, these people are getting on with their lives and learning to accept the bodies they were given—in some cases, even, to celebrate them.

In this department, Wann is leading the pack. She is a hero to many in this crowd for creating a hilarious and sassy underground magazine called *Fat!So?* This hot pink quarterly, based in San Francisco, seems to borrow some of its moxie from that city's gay rights group, Act Up. *Fat!So?* is the 'zine for people who don't apologize for their size. Wann says her mission is to make people ashamed of fat prejudice. Her tactics occasionally extend to acts of civil disobedience, such as when Wann recommended that her readers install in public restrooms rolls of toilet paper printed with fat-positive messages like "waist is a terrible thing to mind." Yet most of the time Wann wages her battle not with guerrilla tactics but with the sly, sharp sword of wit.

For example, take her reaction to the plasticine "glob of fat" that she saw advertised one day in a mail-order catalog. Wann felt compelled to order one, though at first she didn't know why. This wiggly brick was, after all, intended to gross people out—a fat-unfriendly sales pitch if there ever was one. But then it hit her. People are losing pounds of fat all the time. That's what this glob was—a little lost pound of fat—which prompted the mischievous Wann to ask, Where does a pound of fat go when you lose it? Well naturally, it goes on vacation! The Little Lost Lb. o' Fat has since been popping up in tourist spots all over the world and sending back snapshots for *Fat!So?* 's travel section.

The magazine also features a centerfold spread. Not the illicit kind in girlie magazines, but one that manages to shock nonetheless. Under the title "Anatomy Lesson," Wann displays pictures of various fat body parts—chins one month, knees the next, or fleshy triceps that Wann delicately refers to as "arm swag." You never see pictures of this in the conventional media, and the visual impact that Wann's centerfolds have is impressive. The first such spread appeared in the premiere issue—a montage of fat butts. Wann remembers it vividly as part of her "coming out" as a fat person.

It's a funny thing, fat. Even though it is obvious to everyone you meet and may in fact be the only thing people remember about you, admitting that you are heavy or overweight or out-and-out obese is often the hardest thing in the world to do. Though Wann was launching a fat-activist magazine, she struggled with the same feelings. There she was at her local copy store laying out the first issue on a computer. The screen in front of her was filled with pictures of fat butts. Behind her were two glass walls facing onto the street. People kept walking by and stopping and staring at Wann's computer. Two guys finally came in off the street and said they just had to ask her what she was doing. It all made her realize how silly it was that she had been tiptoeing around the subject of fat all her life. Now when people call her fat, Wann agrees with them. Proudly.

Which is why calling obesity a disease rubs Wann the wrong way. "They're trying to find a cure for fatness," she says. "I think the whole pursuit of a cure is offensive." Like most size activists, she believes the current preoccupation with the health risks of obesity is primarily a screen for prejudice. "There's nothing wrong with being fat," Wann writes in the *Fat!So?* manifesto 1, "just like there's nothing wrong with being short or tall, or black or brown. These are facts of identity that cannot and should not be changed. They are birthright. They're beyond aesthetics. They provide the diversity we need to survive."

Such ideas are staples of the size-acceptance movement. Fat activists don't buy the medical argument that obesity is a chronic disease that has statistically been shown to have a substantial impact on life expectancy. They counter that the health consequences of being fat are not easily separated from the way in which health care is delivered to the fat population and the way weight is viewed by fat patients, by doctors, and by society in general. To members of the size-rights community, the problem that most needs to be fought isn't fat itself but peoples' attitudes toward fat.

A Size-Unfriendly World

As an example of those attitudes, activists often refer to an incident that has come to be known in their community as the Chicago Outrage. It revolves around the death of Patricia Mullen, a 31-year-old woman who lived on Chicago's North Side with her three daughters. Mullen was a member of the Chicago Chapter of NAAFA, and she weighed about 500 pounds. On May 7, 1996, she suffered a heart attack and died in her bathroom, where two of her daughters, aged 11 and 7, found her when they came home from school. Shortly thereafter Mullen's niece, Dawn Meschick, notified the police of the death and asked them to take the body to the coroner's office for an autopsy. An officer told Meschick that Mullen was "too fucking fat."

When Meschick persisted, police officers dragged Mullen's naked body into the middle of the living room floor and left it there, with the front door propped open and the curtains not drawn. There Mullen's body lay uncovered for five hours while the officers bellowed crude jokes about its size to a crowd of children who were watching the proceedings. During that time the policemen also made themselves at home in Mullen's house. They listened to music, played with her Nintendo game, and offered food out of her kitchen to passers-by. Neighbors reported a carnival-like atmosphere. They also witnessed the officers jiggling Mullen's body with the toes of their boots and laughing at the effect.

When the coroner's van finally arrived, Mullen's still-naked body was dragged by the ankles up the steps from the basement apartment and across the lawn. The police dropped her at least once along the way, much to their amusement, and then parked her body on the curb. Lee Martindale, a size activist and editor of *Rump Parliament* magazine, reported that at this point a neighbor approached the police, asking them to preserve Mullen's dignity and cover the body with a sheet. The officers responded to the request with curses and threats.

If any punishment was meted out to members of Chicago's finest as a result of the Mullen incident, it was relatively minor. After Mullen's family filed a formal complaint, the Chicago Police Department's Office of Professional Standards investigated. But the results of that investigation were not made public, as is the norm unless an officer is either dismissed or suspended for more than 30 days.

Within the size-acceptance community, the event triggered an outpouring of rage and grief. "In all the years I've been involved in size-rights activism," said Martindale, "and despite the thousands of stories of discrimination and oppression I've experienced or covered or heard, this one hit me hard. . . . I'm not alone in these feelings. Never before have I seen so many people expressing the fear that it could happen to them, that it could happen where they live."

The incident confirmed fat peoples' worst fears that even in death, they cannot escape the barrage of insults that accompanies their weight—the undisguised gestures, the rude comments from strangers, and the harassment from family members under the guise of concern. Anyone who has been the victim of prejudice of any sort can attest that such constant negative input can have a profound effect on both the lives and the health of people who are fat. Ellen Gordon, a NAAFA member from New York, says that if she hadn't had to endure the discrimination and harassment that she did at 150 pounds, she wouldn't be a hundred pounds more today. "Because when you go out in public at a heavy weight you are a different person. It changes you."

To counteract this toxic environment, fat activists strive to create a size-friendly world. Often this involves such seemingly trivial tasks as generating products and services that normal weight people take for granted, like fanny packs with straps that are long enough, airline seat-belt extenders, and extra-large towels. Fat-friendly retailers with names like Big Ass Sportswear and Sweet Cheeks now provide a variety of fashion choices for ample men and women.

Remaking the world to fit the needs of fat people also means creating safe havens where fat people can relax and have a good time, from the size-positive dances put on by Big Sensations in Waltham, Massachusetts, to the Fat Lip Readers Theater in Berkeley, California. Francis White, president of NAAFA since 1991, sees that group's local and national meetings as a place where she doesn't have to "prove to people that she's smarter, faster, funnier" to compensate for her weight. She doesn't have to tell her story to convince them that she's all right.

In some cases, the effort to normalize size has led to some odd dichotomies. The size-acceptance movement has, for example, embraced the word "fat" to describe themselves despite its almost universally negative connotations. They have taken it back in much the same way that some gay groups have taken back the word "queer" because other words simply don't measure up. "Overweight" implies that there is something wrong with being fat. As fat activists are fond of saying, no one is ever described as overheight. "Obesity" is tainted by its association with disease, which runs counter to the size-acceptance movement's view that being fat is a natural human variation.

Yet as a result of this stance, the movement now finds itself in the awkward position of alienating many of the people it would like to attract. Many outside the movement are frightened away by the "f" word. In recent years, this has been the source of some disagreement within NAAFA. Removing "Fat" from the group's title, some leaders argue, might encourage a larger membership. Those who are opposed to making such a change feel it would be a form of surrender to society's "fat phobia" and that it would legitimize the self-hatred felt already by so many fat people.

Size Rights

Whether or not they succeed in reclaiming the language, to truly create a size-friendly environment fat activists are also working to reclaim the basic civil rights that fat people are routinely denied. NAAFA has fought this battle on many fronts, but it has placed particular emphasis on the issue of health care. One of the most important health issues for obese people, according to NAAFA, is the fact that many fat people do not receive adequate preventive health care, and they shun treatment even after a medical problem arises. This, size activists say, is a direct result of prejudicial medical treatment and harassment by health care professionals over the years.

Surveys of the medical community have repeatedly provided evidence of this size prejudice. In a 1969 survey, doctors rated obese people as ugly, awkward, and weak-willed. A more recent study, published in 1987, demonstrated that an aversion to heavy patients persisted. The study group consisted of 318 family practice physicians. Two-thirds of them said that they believed their obese patients lacked self-control. Over a third described obese people as "lazy" and "sad."

Obesity research has been making the headlines more frequently during the 1990s, and it is possible that such widespread attention to the biological causes of obesity has made doctors more sensitive to size issues. Up-to-date surveys are not available. But the group of physicians that would seem to be best equipped to address the medical needs of fat patients, that is, the obesity researchers themselves, have drawn particular wrath from the size-rights community.

Activists are well-versed in the multiple conflicts of interest that plague obesity researchers. Many of these medical professionals are paid consultants to commercial weight-loss programs, to manufacturers of diet products, or to diet drug companies. Obesity conferences are routinely underwritten by pharmaceutical firms, and many obesity researchers conduct clinical trials for new diet drugs. Such financial ties indicate the enormous economic stake that obesity researchers have in seeing expanded forms of obesity treatment applied to more and more Americans.

This isn't to say that size activists would put an end to medical research on obesity. NAAFA supports and encourages research into the causes of obesity. But its leaders know that the value of the results depends to a large extent on how they are applied. Obesity researchers, says NAAFA executive director Sally Smith, are too eager to find a quick fix for fatness instead of looking for ways to help fat people stay healthy.

To redress these problems, NAAFA has issued a Declaration of the Rights of Fat People in Health Care. Some of its tenets are so fundamental that they illustrate how fully the medical profession has failed to address the needs of large people, even as the numbers of those people gradually eclipse the population of people who are lean. Fat people have the right, NAAFA asserts, "to adequate physical accommodations, equipment and testing facilities in the health care setting." By this the group means that obese patients should routinely have access to items like exam tables that are large enough, gowns that can cover a large body, blood pressure cuffs of the right size to give accurate readings, and personnel who are trained to draw blood from a fat person's arm without unnecessary discomfort.

Although the lack of these elements could conceivably be attributed to benign neglect and could be readily rectified by the medical profession, NAAFA claims another basic health care right that puts it in direct conflict with the average doctor's view of obesity as a condition that demands medical treatment. Fat people have the right, says NAAFA, "to refuse participation in weight loss programs of all kinds, including diets, surgery, aversive psychological conditioning, and chemical regimes, without jeopardizing access to other treatment and care."

NAAFA's position is that permanent weight loss is impossible for most fat people to achieve, and dieting only makes people fatter; therefore doctors should quit trying to put people on diets, and they should never insist that a patient lose weight prior to treatment even if the weight increases the chance that a medical procedure, like surgery, will go badly. Indeed the antidieting sentiment runs so strong within the size-acceptance community that NAAFA's Sally Smith has called for a federal labeling and advertising act that would ban radio and television commercials for weight-loss diets and products. Smith says that such an act, modeled on the 1971 Federal Cigarette Labeling and Advertising Act, would help end the social stigma and discrimination against fat people.

Of all the weight treatments used by both doctors and patients over the years, dieting has been the most popular. In the light of this legacy, Smith's goal of a federal act still seems quite radical. Yet there are a number of indications that the popularity of dieting has begun to wane. National diet programs like Nutri/System and Jenny Craig have seen their annual revenues plunge in recent years, and market analysts are attributing the decline to a growing belief that diets don't work. Medical professionals have also begun to suggest that too much emphasis has been placed on restriction dieting and weight loss as the keys to health, and not enough on activity, weight maintenance, and metabolic fitness.

What Is Real?

Yet even as size activists have watched dieting fall slowly out of favor, they have witnessed the rebirth of an age-old enemy. "I think the current challenge that fat people will face is a whole new generation of diet drugs," says Marilyn Wann. Most members of the size-acceptance movement consider the right to not subject themselves to another round of dashed hopes and intolerable health risks as fundamental. "We're determined that we're not going to pay again for drugs that harm us rather than help us," says size activist Lynn McAfee.

McAfee, like many of her fellow activists, speaks from first-hand experience with the earlier amphetamine diet pills. She was put on these drugs at the age of 6. "I'm an amphetamine child," she says matter-of-factly. "So that really challenged my sense of what's real—when you're speeding on amphetamines when you're 6 years old, having altered-consciousness experiences." Now in her late forties, McAfee looks back on the impact of those drugged-up days and says that the search for "what is real" has been a theme in her life ever since.

It motivated her to take a job as a page in the medical library at the College of Physicians of Philadelphia during her early twenties. "I took it," says McAfee, "partly because I thought, This is the chance to find out the perfect diet. Obviously there's something I don't know and I'll find out the secret. So I worked there for three years and I read every single article—several thousand journals over three years. And I just found 95- to 98-percent failure rates. I kept waiting for it to be announced—that it wasn't just you that was the problem—and it never was. I asked a doctor why and he said, 'Well, nobody wants to discourage people from losing weight.' I thought, Well, that's really nuts."

Shortly after that, Cass Elliot of the Mamas and the Papas died. For McAfee, this was a watershed event in her career as a size activist. She was incensed by the rumors that Elliot, one of the few fat women in the public eye, had choked to death on a ham sandwich—rumors that were started by a flippant remark to that effect from Elliot's own physician. The comment was quoted in Elliot's *New York Times* obituary.

In fact, an autopsy of the singer by two British doctors later showed that she had died of a heart attack. Once this news came out, McAfee could no longer contain her anger. She strapped on a black armband and led a candlelight march directly into a crowd that had gathered for a Women's Day celebration. Before this audience, she let loose a fervent protest of Elliot's treatment. The experience stirred something inside McAfee; she has been working as a size activist for the quarter of a century since.

Yet McAfee's feelings about diet drugs differ in some fundamental ways from those of her fellow activists. Rather than seeing the new drugs as an enemy, McAfee believes in their potential. She believes in working to achieve their potential by interacting with obesity researchers, drug companies, and government agencies. In her own way McAfee is working toward the health rights of fat people so that they will not be shortchanged by the medical system.

McAfee says she understands why her fellow activists tend to be suspicious of attempts to treat them. "Obesity researchers for many, many decades have had extremely rigid rhetoric," she says. "The whole 'fat is evil' kind of thinking. Fat has to be fought. We have to fight ourselves and fight our bodies. . . . The researchers say obesity is bad and all fat people are diseased. And size-acceptance people say, No, we're not, none of that is true, because an extreme response engenders an extreme response."

"Size-acceptance people want to see that fat is not the cause of everything bad in the world," McAfee continues. "But by doing that, it's really hard not to sort of go overboard, you know? And I don't want to do that right now. I want to keep myself open to thinking, Yeah, you know, fat people do have different bodies." If it is possible for researchers to understand those differences and develop ways to circumvent them, McAfee is all for it.

In 1991 she formed the Council on Size and Weight Discrimination. She now spends her days on the phone with drug company scientists, doctors, legislators, and journalists. She has attended every meeting of the FDA's Endocrinologic and Metabolic Drugs Advisory Committee, which reviews new anti-obesity drug applications. In 1997 the NIH Task Force on Prevention and Treatment of Obesity invited her to be on the planning committee for a five-year study that they are launching. The study will attempt to determine whether people are really healthier if they lose weight.

In all these roles, McAfee functions as a watchdog and a spokesperson for the needs of fat people. She has urged the makers of Meridia to acknowledge that their customers are going to be fat and that therefore the advertising for this product should include fat-positive images. She has publicly chastised the FDA for requiring thorough, long-term testing of antiobesity medications *after* they are approved, instead of before. She has criticized individual researchers for throwing their influence behind antiobesity medications with such intolerable side-effects that the drugs are an insult to the people who take them. McAfee may be interacting with the people who develop drugs, but she is still very much an outsider.

As a 500-pound woman, McAfee grew accustomed to being an outsider long ago. She considers it a reasonable price for the opportunity to remind drug developers exactly who they are working to help. It is important, she believes, for scientists to step away from their molecules and their theories occasionally to see their work through the eyes a former amphetamine child like herself. "I say to obesity researchers sometimes, You know, it's all your fault that I'm really on your case like this, because all I ever cared about was what's reality, what's true, because it never was what my experience was. But that's what we really have to look at. What is real? What is peoples' experience? That has to drive the science."

SEVEN

In Deference to Difference

**INDIVIDUAL
VARIABILITY AND
THE FUTURE OF
WEIGHT CONTROL**

"Isaid, 'Hold on a minute. You're telling me about a virus killing chickens and then you're saying that they have *more* fat?'" Nikhil Dhurandhar recalled. A nutritionist from Bombay, Dhurandhar's voice rises a notch when he talks about the conversation he had several years ago. One of his colleagues in India, veterinary pathologist Sharad Ajinkya, had been puzzling over a virus that was killing flocks of chickens in the Bombay area. Ajinkya made a casual remark to Dhurandhar that while doing autopsies of some of the infected birds, he noticed that they had a thick layer of fat around their bellies.

"Why is that?" Dhurandhar pressed him. Ajinkya didn't know the answer. "Well, can you verify it?" That Ajinkya could do. He had seen enough dead chickens in his day to know that the fat was out of the ordinary and that this virus, one of a family called adenoviruses, was the cause. When the two men took 20 chickens and injected them with the virus, they showed that it was indeed the adenovirus that was making these animals obese.

Dhurandhar couldn't help but wonder whether people could possibly catch an obesity virus the way these chickens had. At the time of the experiment, he was treating obese patients in his Bombay clinic. "Just for the heck of it," he said, "I looked at their blood to look for antibodies to this avian adenovirus." Antibodies would imply that the patients had either been infected with this chicken virus or with a human virus that was remarkably similar.

Dhurandhar didn't really expect to find anything. He knew that avian adenoviruses weren't supposed to infect people. At least that had been the assumption for decades, since bird viruses in general don't have the structures they need to infect human cells. Historically, incidents of infections jumping from birds to people were almost unheard of—until the Hong Kong bird flu broke out in May 1997.

That virus killed 6 people and made 18 more sick before the Hong Kong government ordered all of the chickens in the country slaughtered to prevent a pandemic. The outbreak shattered the notion that people were safe from avian viruses. When Dhurandhar followed his curiosity with the chicken obesity virus, he gleaned hints of the same phenomenon. Out of the 52 obese patients whose blood he sampled, 10 had antibodies against the virus.

Dhurandhar also found one other piece of evidence that convinced him that the chicken virus was associated with human obesity. In the birds that grew obese, Dhurandhar noticed that the levels of cholesterol and triglycerides, the form that fat takes in the bloodstream, were lower than in the normal, uninfected birds. This was a particularly odd result. Obese animals as well as obese people usually have higher than normal levels of cholesterol and triglycerides. Yet in the obese patients who showed antibodies to the virus, Dhurandhar saw the same odd set of symptoms. The people were obese but without the dangerous levels of cholesterol and triglycerides that usually accompany that condition. "So after that, I thought, This is too important a finding to let go," Dhurandhar recalls. "I closed my practice and I came here."

"Here" is the University of Wisconsin in Madison, where Dhurandhar has been collaborating with Richard Atkinson. One of the senior members of the obesity research community, Atkinson has been interested in obesity viruses ever since he read a 1982 paper in *Science* magazine that described the first such virus ever discovered in animals—one that made 15 percent of the mice it infected obese. Since Atkinson's field is human obesity, he felt the subject was too far afield to pursue. But when Dhurandhar connected the chicken virus to obesity in people, Atkinson said, "I knew I really needed to get this guy in the lab."

Although Dhurandhar garnered a fellowship and funds to pursue a human obesity virus, there was a hitch. There are laws against bringing a virus across foreign borders. Poultry farmers in the United States could not afford to have their chickens accidentally exposed to a lethal virus from India. If this virus could also infect people and make them fat, then all the more reason to keep it out. There are already enough illnesses hitching rides with transcontinental travelers without adding an obesity virus to the mix. Dhurandhar had to start his research in the United States more or less from scratch.

To find an obesity virus in the United States, Dhurandhar and Atkinson turned to a bank of existing adenoviruses. The approach was a long shot, but they had to hope that some American scientist had already seen and catalogued an obesity virus without knowing what it was. In particular, the researchers went looking for a human virus, not a chicken one, since they wanted to see its effects in people, not birds. They searched for either a chicken virus that had mutated so that it could infect people or a human virus that had begun to infect chickens. Either way, it might show up among the array of viruses already known in people.

Their first choice was a virus called AD36. "We had nothing to go by," said Dhurandhar. "We were given a list of about 50 different types of human adenoviruses that one can buy here in this country, and we had to choose one that causes obesity when there was no mention about it in the description of the virus. So we kind of looked for similarities with the virus that we worked with before, in India. And also this particular virus was isolated from a diabetic girl initially. Diabetes and obesity are closely related, so we thought there might be a link. Not great science there, but what else could we do?"

In their search for antibodies to AD36 in the blood of obese patients, Dhurandhar and Atkinson struck gold.

They found that about 15 percent of the obese people they tested had antibodies, whereas none of the lean people did. What's more, those who had antibodies to AD36 also had unusually low levels of cholesterol and triglycerides, just as Dhurandhar had seen with the Indian chicken virus, which raised the possibility that AD36 may even be the same virus that was seen in India. As yet it's too soon for the researchers to say. These two viruses and perhaps other obesity viruses may simply cause this specific set of symptoms in both animals and people because they strike at the same part of the weight-control system.

The researchers are now in the midst of a flurry of experiments to sort out such questions and determine whether they have found what they were looking for—a virus that infects people and makes them fat. Much more evidence is needed, because the fact that obese people have antibodies to the virus doesn't necessarily prove that it caused their obesity. Dhurandhar can show that the virus definitely causes obesity in chickens. He injected them with it and watched as the chickens grew in size. But he obviously can't do that experiment with people. People won't volunteer to get an injection of an obesity virus.

The human obesity virus, while plausible, has yet to be proven. As some virologists have pointed out, obese people may be more susceptible to this virus for reasons we don't yet understand. For now, most obesity researchers are simply shrugging their shoulders and waiting for more evidence. Still, they don't reject the theory outright. The idea that a virus could cause obesity sounds a lot less outlandish when you realize that in recent years viruses have been associated with a host of human diseases that we never would have thought possible. Viruses are implicated in several types of cancer, atherosclerosis, and mood disorders like depression and obsessive-compulsive disorder. Now a handful of viruses have been shown to cause obesity in animals, and that lends weight to the case for a human obesity virus. Besides AD36 and the original chicken virus, three other animal obesity viruses have been discovered. If animals can get fat from a virus, why not people?

A Nationwide Epidemic

Pursuing this obesity virus idea has led the researchers to pose an even more radical theory. The number of people in the United States who fit the clinical definition of obese (a body mass index of 30 or more) stayed at the relatively constant level of about 14 percent of the population between 1960 and 1980. But then in a single decade it rose to 22.5 percent. What if the recent jump in obesity wasn't caused by our sedentary habits or our fast-food culture or one of the other often-cited environmental influences? What if it was a result of a virus that had swept through the population and caused those whom it infected to become susceptible to weight gain?

"I ask people," Dhurandhar said, "'Can you tell me what happened in the last ten years that changed the prevalence of obesity so dramatically?' And they say, 'Oh, people are exercising less.' But then was that different ten years ago? Were there no McDonalds and Burger Kings ten years ago? There is little that can explain this big jump in the prevalence. So we're just speculating here. Could it be due to a virus?"

It's an interesting idea to ponder—tentative though it may be. Adenoviruses usually cause mild respiratory infections in people. But it isn't as if you would get a cold one day and become obese the next. The effect on weight would be more gradual—an increased susceptibility, a tendency to eat a bit more, say, or burn calories a little slower. How could a virus have that effect? The early studies on obesity viruses in animals give us a hint. Researchers studying the mouse virus detected it in areas of the animal's brain that regulate eating and body weight for up to six weeks after the animals were infected. One theory was that the mouse obesity virus worked by causing damage to these brain regions. Even after the virus was out of the system, the damage seemed to cause permanent changes in the animals' ability to maintain a stable weight.

Whether AD36 acts in the same way is still unknown. Dhurandhar looked at the brains of mice infected with the virus and he saw no damage. His early assessment was that this virus probably does not affect the brain negatively. But the body's weight-control apparatus has many components and a virus could cause damage in any of many different parts of that system. The impact of the virus could also be quite gradual; over the course of a decade the effect could be substantial.

Atkinson says, "I think it's a little bit too incredible to believe that all obesity is due to adenoviruses." He points to the fact that antibodies show up in only a fraction of the obese patients the researchers have looked at. But he and Dhurandhar suggest that obesity viruses might explain a portion of the rapid worldwide increases in obesity.

Why Are People Fat?

We could add viruses to a long list of causes of obesity. If any single theme has emerged from research on obesity over the last decade, it is that no one simple explanation exists for why people get fat. Health experts have put forth a number of possible explanations for our recent weight gain, from city planning that discourages exercise to high-fat diets to stress. Every one of these factors undoubtedly has contributed to the rise in American obesity. Work on the genetics of weight control has also shown that in order for those environmental influences to take hold, we have to have obesity programmed in our genes. Indeed, it now appears that the genetic causes of obesity are even more numerous than the environmental ones.

Researchers once hoped that there might be just a handful of genes that could account for a susceptibility to weight gain. Finding them and tackling the condition of obesity would then have been a relatively straightforward process. Over the last decade however, researchers have come to accept that such a scenario was too good to be true. "It's quite clear that it's not due to a few genetic problems," says Atkinson, emphasizing the word *few*.

As evidence, Atkinson refers to an update on the search for obesity genes that the Canadian researcher Claude Bouchard publishes every year in the journal

Obesity Research. In the most recent update, Bouchard identified 75 genes and gene markers that are in some way associated with human obesity. "It's simplistic to do it this way," Atkinson says, "but if you think about all the combinations and permutations of those 75 genes, there are going to be dozens, hundreds, thousands of different *kinds* of obesity."

The way the genes come together is different in each of us. In one person, susceptibility to weight gain might be caused by a handful of different gene-controlled factors: a gut that is slow to signal fullness, muscles that need remarkably little fuel to keep them going, perhaps even some damage to the brain's satiety center as a result of a viral infection. It's rare that we think about our internal organs as having so much variety. One pancreatic gland seems pretty much like any other. But consider for a moment the genetic variety that we see every day when we look at the faces of the people around us.

We are all born with the same basic facial features—eyes, nose, and mouth. Yet they somehow come together in a way that is different for each of us. Our nose may come from one parent, our eyes from the other. For our mouth we may have to reach way back into the family lineage to find a replica. Distinguishing us from brothers or sisters who might have the same combination of features are the subtler details of complexion, eye color, hairline, the shape of an ear, or a peculiar wrinkle between our eyebrows. All these superficial traits contribute to our individuality and make it possible to pick out an individual from the other 6 billion people on earth.

We're unique on the inside too—not just in the heart-warming sense that everyone is special in their own way but also literally. From our brains to our guts to our pancreatic enzymes, our bodies each have their own characteristic style in the way in which weight is controlled. By recognizing these differences, scientists are edging us toward a new and more useful definition of what it means to be fat.

Slow Metabolisms, Fast Metabolisms

One of the researchers who has consistently called attention to the individual nature of weight control over the last decade is Eric Ravussin, a visiting scientist at a branch of the National Institute of Diabetes and Digestive and Kidney Diseases in Phoenix, Arizona. The Phoenix lab is devoted to the study of the Pima Indians, a group of native Americans that have a high rate of obesity and diabetes. Ravussin has been exploring the metabolism of this population. Is there something about the way the Pimas' bodies use energy that has made them particularly susceptible to weight gain? Can this help explain obesity in the rest of the nation?

In a decade of work, Ravussin has uncovered some fascinating differences in how people burn energy and how the differences contribute to weight gain. Some obese people, for example, tend to burn fat relatively slowly or they fail to increase the amount of fat they burn even when the fat content in their diet goes up. As a result, these people gain weight more readily than most of us when they are exposed to a high-fat diet. Ravussin has found that other people who are susceptible to obesity show very little of what he calls spontaneous physical activity—fidgeting, toe tapping, hair twirling. Even though these actions may be unconscious, they make a substantial contribution to overall energy use.

To uncover these aspects of energy burning, Ravussin measured the metabolic rates of hundreds of people of all weights and backgrounds. The experience provided him with an enormous range of data on peoples' metabolic rates. It also led to Ravussin's realization that even within a fairly homogenous population like the Pimas, metabolic rates can vary widely.

In one study of more than 500 Pima volunteers, Ravussin and his colleague Pietro Tataranni analyzed resting metabolism, or how much energy the body expends just to maintain basic functions like temperature control and involuntary muscle activity. The researchers gathered this information using a clear plastic, ventilated hood that is specially designed for the task. The hood fits snugly around a subject's neck and looks like something out of a viral scare movie. It continuously draws air in and siphons it off while the test subject lies motionless and awake for 40 minutes. During that time, researchers measure how much oxygen the test subject consumes and how much carbon dioxide he or she respires. By doing this, they can determine how much energy the person is expending. That's because whenever people transform the energy they get from food into heat or muscular work, they use oxygen in the process. A quick calculation provides researchers with the number of calories the subject uses over the course of a day—the resting metabolic rate.

Ravussin and Tataranni found that resting metabolic rates varied within their volunteers from 1067 to 3015 calories per day—a threefold difference in the amount of food people could burn in a given 24-hour period. Of course, there are a lot of different factors that go into a person's metabolism, and these account for some of the variation. For example, the bigger you are, the more energy you use to keep all your cells running. Body composition is also a major factor. Lean tissue burns about four times the energy at rest that fat tissue burns. To a lesser extent, gender and age also play a role in our metabolic rates. Women, as a rule, have lower rates than men, and older people burn less fuel than younger ones, though most of the variations among age groups can be explained by differences in body composition. Yet even when Ravussin eliminated these factors, he still found a large range of metabolic rates within the population.

Some people seem to be blessed with a higher than average metabolism and others have just the opposite. This is something that people who struggle with weight control have been saying for years, and Ravussin is well aware that most people think they know whether their metabolism is fast or slow, usually based on their weight. "Most of the obese patients you see, they'll tell you, 'Oh, I have something wrong with my metabolism,'" says Ravussin with a trace of the accent from his native Switzerland. "And you know, personally I believe that something is wrong. But it may not be metabolic rate."

Contrary to what many people think, he says, the only way to know your metabolic rate is to measure it directly. And when Ravussin has measured rates he has found that a slow metabolism doesn't necessarily go hand in hand with obesity.

A low metabolic rate can, of course, contribute to weight gain. Ravussin cowrote a study several years ago that showed that a person's resting metabolic rate was a good predictor of how much weight he or she would gain over a four-year period. But Ravussin and his colleagues also found that not everyone in this study who had a slow metabolism gained weight. What's more, even among those people who gained more than 22 pounds, the researchers said that only 40 percent of the weight gain could be accounted for by the differences in metabolism. Other factors, like food consumption or daily activity, had to make up the difference.

This means that even though many people with low metabolic rates are prone to weight gain, you can't really look at people who are overweight or obese and say anything about their metabolism or what role it plays in their weight. People with the same physical characteristics— same weight, same height, same basic shape—may nevertheless burn vastly different amounts of energy each day just to maintain these characteristics. "I mean you don't need a rocket scientist to know that among the obese . . . there are some major differences between these people," says Ravussin. And recognizing this is important, he says, "because if the causes of obesity are different, the treatment should be different."

Tailoring Treatment

When it comes to weight, it has long been our habit to group heavy people together as if they all suffered from the same condition and should all respond to the same cure. Every diet and exercise program is pitched as the one-size-fits-all remedy for weight problems. Physicians who treat obesity have applied psychotherapy and, later, behavior therapy to everyone. It's no wonder that efforts to treat obesity have had such an abysmally poor success rate over the last half-century. That's the explanation favored by Colorado obesity researcher James Hill. "I think we took a group of subjects who are really apples and oranges and we didn't know that," he says. "We treated them the same and we probably got different responses and we got no result."

Human variety influences the effectiveness of obesity treatment. Nowhere is this more evident than when you look at how the range of metabolic rates affects the standard medical approach to obesity treatment: an eating program. You might consider yourself lucky if you went looking for treatment for a weight problem and you found a doctor who took the time to calculate your resting metabolic rate and then assigned you to an eating regimen tailored to your energy needs. But the practice among many physicians who treat obesity is to estimate energy expenditure based on a person's height, weight, age, and sex. The problem is, such calculations can give figures that are way off the mark.

University of Pennsylvania obesity researcher Gary Foster showed in a study done a decade ago that energy predictions are only modestly related to actual measurements. Out of a sample of 80 obese women, he took 5 with virtually the same predicted resting energy expenditure and showed that their measured rates ranged from 27 percent lower than expected to 23 percent higher. "A typical six-month, 1,200 kcal/day treatment program," Foster and his coauthors wrote, "would result in weight losses of 10, 18, 26, 32, and 37 kilograms [22 to 81 pounds]."

An even more surprising example of how human variety impacts treatment lies in the one health recommendation that you'd think would be ironclad—the beneficial effects of exercise. One of the startling results to come out of research over the last decade is that exercise also has vastly different effects in different people.

In a conference on exercise and obesity held in 1994, one of the chairmen of the meeting, Claude Bouchard, chose to devote his talk to this topic. Bouchard is the researcher who has been taking measurements of Quebec family members for the last 20 years. He's the world expert on genetics and fitness. He began his talk with some widely known statistics on the effect a regular exercise program can have on a group of sedentary people. After three to four months of endurance exercise, for example, young adults can experience a 20- to 25-percent increase in their VO2max—a measure of cardiorespiratory fitness that is usually determined by a treadmill test. "This is commonly observed," Bouchard said, "and is recognized to the point that it has become one of the exercise science dogmas."

But having lulled his audience into a sense of confidence with statistics that most of them already knew, he then reminded them of something else that they probably knew but often forgot. Such figures are only average values, and the averages mask the vast range of responses to exercise that exists within the population. "In reality," Bouchard said, "most people who are training under similar conditions do not register such gains."

Bouchard then proceeded to give examples of the many ways he and his colleagues can measure a person's physical response to exercise along with the ranges they have seen. As he did, a startling fact became apparent. Just as there are some people who show great improvements in fitness from regular exercise, there are others who seem to show no response at all. When Bouchard put a group of 47 young men on a training program for 15 to 20 weeks, in one example, he found that some showed 100 percent improvement in their VO2max, while others showed almost no change. He has seen the same lack of response in other measurements of how people adapt to exercise, such as heart size, muscle fiber size, and how much work they can perform in a 90-minute interval. "We believe it is quite remarkable," he said, "that for all the determinants that have been considered in a series of investigations performed in our laboratory, one can find nonresponders even after 20 weeks of regular exercise at a frequency of five times a week over the last several weeks of the program."

Naturally, Bouchard would like to know what kind of person doesn't respond to exercise. For now, his research hasn't produced any obvious type of person. Most of his studies on this topic were done with young adults, 18 to 30 years old. Since there were nonresponders in these groups, it doesn't appear that the lack of response is a result of aging. Similarly, both men and women can be nonresponders. The condition simply seems to be part of the range of human diversity.

What is even more confounding to researchers about nonresponders is that at the moment, knowing that someone has this trait still leaves open the question of what to do with the information. It isn't like knowing that someone has a slow metabolism. There, the best strategy to maintain a healthy weight would be to limit calorie intake to what they can burn in a day. But it's hard to prescribe a treatment strategy for people who show no response to exercise since it is nearly impossible to determine if these people are deriving any benefit from exercise at all.

Some of Bouchard's research touched on this problem. He looked at the impact that exercise had on risk factors for weight-related diseases like diabetes and cardiovascular disease. In one study, a dozen young adult males rode stationary bikes two hours a day for 22 straight days. When Bouchard looked at the effects of this exercise on cholesterol levels, blood fat, and insulin levels, he noted differences of as much as fivefold between individuals in the study group. The broad range of effects indicates that in some people, exercise has a much greater impact on risk factors and, by extension, health than in others. Still, that isn't quite the same as looking at the long-term death rates of nonresponders to see if the ones who exercise live any longer than the ones who don't. And it doesn't begin to touch on the psychological benefits of activity—the feelings of control and self-esteem. Obesity researchers simply do not know if there are people who *don't* benefit from exercise.

Exercise booster Stephen Blair, who spearheaded the idea that people could be fit and fat, concedes the possibility that activity isn't the secret of life for everyone. "Human beings vary on every single trait that anyone's thought to measure," he says. "So I think it would be reasonable to assume that some people get relatively more benefit than others, benefit in terms of health protection, with the same dose of exercise." But since no one knows how large that benefit is, he adds, "you're right back to that statement of the American College of Sports Medicine and the CDC, that people who do at least moderate amounts of activity seem to be a whole lot better off as a group."

Weight Control of the Future

Our understanding of the many ways that different bodies control weight is still in its infancy. Nonetheless, we now face a future in which we will be able to characterize many different types of obesity. With each new piece of the weight-control puzzle researchers set in place, they are gradually changing the way we see weight treatment.

Scientists envision a day when we will be able to go into a weight-control center or a doctor's office and have a complete workup. Analyses of metabolism are already becoming more commonplace. The tony Canyon Ranch spa, with locations in Massachusetts' Berkshire hills and in Tucson, Arizona, will measure your metabolism for $400. All it takes is a few minutes in a plastic hood similar to the one used in Eric Ravussin's lab. A simple blood test is all that's necessary to measure the levels of many of the newly discovered biochemical compounds like leptin that are involved in weight control. A test for an obesity virus may even be part of the picture if the research of Atkinson and Dhurandhar pans out. Diagnosing someone's susceptibility to obesity, perhaps even before the weight is gained, is the future of weight control.

The result will be no more one-size-fits-all remedies. From an individual weight-control profile, a doctor may be able to gauge what has contributed to weight gain and what approach to losing weight will give the best response. He or she may prescribe an individually tailored diet or activity program. Knowing a person's weight traits will probably have the greatest impact, however, on the pharmacology of weight control—not only on which types of drugs will become available but also on how they will be used.

People are different, and antiobesity drugs have very different effects on them. This can be said of most drug therapies. It is nothing out of the ordinary—only a lesson that we have had to learn about weight-control drugs as we move toward treating obesity as a physiological condition. In practice, this means not only that weight control drugs will cause serious side effects in a fraction of users, but that in some people the drugs will have no effect at all.

Even in the short time that Redux was on the market in the United States, its varied effects were apparent. Stories of people who lost 30 or 40 pounds on the drug fueled the rush for prescriptions. But just as there were some people who lost weight very successfully, there were others who experienced no reduction at all. The weight-loss figure obesity researchers often associated with Redux—10 percent of initial body weight—was in fact an average that concealed a much broader range of effects. The same variety of effects can be found in people who have used the antiobesity drug, Meridia. Meridia works to suppress appetite by maintaining the levels of the brain chemicals serotonin and norepinephrine. About 10 percent of Meridia users do not lose weight no matter how long they take the drug. And 4 to 10 percent of its users experience potentially lethal increases in blood pressure, while the effect on the remainder of users is negligible.

Doctors are still too ignorant of how the weight-control system works to figure out which drugs will work for whom and which drugs will not. Up to now, there hasn't been a wide variety of diet drugs from which to choose. As a result, we have been taking what fat activist Lynn McAfee calls the "Prozac approach" to weight-loss drugs. In other words, when a drug becomes available, everybody takes it, and if it works, they needed it. As more and more antiobesity drugs become available, however, industry watchers like McAfee believe that the need for scientists and drug manufacturers to give doctors good information about individuals' drug responses will be crucial. "That's my main issue when you look at the future," she says. "I don't want us to have to take every single drug that comes down the pipeline. Particularly for this future leptin generation, neuropeptide Y stuff—I want them to develop testing so that they can look at levels of a chemical in our bodies and say, You're a quart low on this, you're a little high on that."

Obesity researchers put it in slightly more technical terms, but they are thinking along the same lines. Asked to speculate on how the latest genetic discoveries might be put to use, David West, at the Pennington Biomedical Research Center, replied that once researchers know a few of the major genes that contribute to obesity, they might be able to diagnose which versions of those genes a person is carrying, and that could influence drug selection. "You could then screen people and say, 'You're going to respond to drug X but this person over here is not going to respond so we need to find another therapy,'" he said. "I think that's clearly a possibility."

Similar screening tests are already being developed for drugs that target a multitude of conditions besides obesity. In the emerging and controversial field of pharmacogenomics, a handful of companies specializing in gene research are creating diagnostic programs that promise to predict whether patients' genetic profiles are a good match for a particular drug therapy. Such diagnostic tests, though they have not yet reached the mass market, are generating widespread interest among pharmaceutical companies as well as individual doctors.

For now people have to resort to trial and error to figure out whether a weight-control drug will work for them. Their doctors may try prescribing them one drug and then, if that doesn't work, try them on another, in much the same way physicians routinely treat their patients with high blood pressure. Yet even with this scenario, people who take diet drugs can benefit from some crude diagnostic tests that take individual responses into account.

It is quite clear to researchers who have studied the effects of Meridia, for example, that people who will not benefit from this drug can be identified very early in treatment. Users who fail to lose 1 percent of their body weight after taking the drug for four weeks will never be able to lose weight with the drug. Similarly, patients who are likely to experience dangerous spikes in blood pressure can be identified within the first four weeks of treatment. Knowing this, physicians can promptly withdraw their patients from the drug and minimize its potential for harm.

EIGHT

Waddling Towards Bethlehem

IN THE MEANTIME, WHAT SHOULD I DO ABOUT MY WEIGHT?

Every year on the last Saturday in August people gather in the tiny, rural community of Crooked River Ranch, Oregon, for an unusual event: the Short Fat Guys and Gals Road Race. "The race has three rules," says the event's founder, a man who calls himself Crooked River Mitch. "Rule number one is that you must be under seven feet tall in order to qualify as short. If you're seven foot one we're going to call you six foot thirteen so you can qualify anyway. The second rule is that your waist measurement must be at least four and a half inches greater than your inseam. If it's not, we have a pair of scissors."

Mitch begins to chuckle as he tells me the rules. His laugh comes booming over the telephone line like a pumping handshake and a warm slap on the back. He dreamed up this race over a decade ago, and, as his rules imply, it is a race in name only. No one actually runs. In fact, Mitch hates that word. The race is one mile, all downhill, and entrants are required to stop halfway through the course to swallow a free hot dog and a beverage (usually beer). After this pit stop, the entrants then have to come to a halt again 50 feet short of the finish line and wait for everyone to catch up before crossing, which means there are never any winners or losers in this race; every year it's a dead heat.

The only real competition is in who can get across the finish line with the most style and showmanship. That's why Mitch emphasizes rule number three: cheating is encouraged. In 1994 he "raced" to the finish line seated on a flatbed truck complete with tables, chairs, and waitress service. The next year, Mitch strapped saddlebags onto a goat and tried to make it carry his beer and him as well.

At 6 feet 1 inch and 245 pounds, Mitch is more than even the most accommodating goat can bear. The animal threw him, and the two finished the race on hoof and foot. Mitch took it with his usual Falstaffian air. After all, he invented this race to poke fun at the major marathons in the world. "See, all of those guys think they're super athletes," he says. "But those of us in the Short Fat Guys and Gals Road Race, we know we're super athletes. We don't have to prove anything. So we go out and just have fun."

While those of us who are concerned about excess pounds wait for the science of weight control to catch up to its potential, there are a few things we can do for our health. Mitch, in his mischievous way, has put his finger on a few of them—not because a diet of hot dogs and beer is particularly healthy nor because there is some weight-loss magic that comes from riding a goat, but simply because in the midst of a cultural barrage of thin mania, Mitch seems to have fashioned a good-humored response.

First, Mitch knows that a little junk food washed down with a few beers isn't going to kill anyone. Our culture makes it easy to convince ourselves that by focusing on what we eat and what we weigh, we are taking an active role in promoting our health. Yet again and again, scientific research has shown that one of the first lines of defense against weight problems is getting over an obsession with dieting and thinness. That doesn't mean that we should all go out and organize pie-eating contests in our hometowns. But fighting against the cultural forces that entice us to fixate on food and at the same time pressure us to look svelte takes a little active effort of the sort Mitch demonstrates.

The next time you hear a phrase like "sinfully delicious," pause to consider the true implications of dividing foods into "good" and "bad." When you see some actress and wish your body looked more like hers, remind yourself that her appearance is the product of a team of trainers, stylists, surgeons, airbrush artists and body doubles. Count your blessings that you are free to focus on something besides the shape of your hindquarters. And if you should hear about a great new diet, ask yourself which is really the best thing for your body, a regimen that recommends vast quantities of meat or a reasonable volume of a wide variety of foods.

Mitch also knows that a leisurely stroll down a hill followed by a night of revelry at the after-race celebration is a far cry better for his health than lying on the couch watching Saturday's football lineup. No one would call what Mitch and his fellow racers are doing vigorous exercise. Even calling it moderate exercise is a stretch. But what the Short Fat Guys and Gals are not doing is being inactive.

In the race to a healthy weight, we would all do well to incorporate some sort of exercise into our daily routines—preferably at least 30 minutes of continuous and slightly challenging activity. But in the spirit of Mitch's race, a little cheating should also be encouraged. If you feel like window shopping instead of lifting weights at the gym, there's no need to beat yourself up about it. The point is to stay active in whatever manner suits you best. In the long run, the activity you enjoy doing is far more likely to get done than the one that seems like a chore.

Junior Knows Best

Perhaps the most important reason for letting go of our sedentary habits and our infatuation with dieting is not so much to get our own weights in line but to prevent our children from absorbing our unhealthy attitudes. On a recent flight to Phoenix, a woman seated behind me was making funny faces at my 1-year-old son. "What do you do when he doesn't eat?" she asked me, after remarking on his beefy appearance. She told me that she had a daughter about the same age who was a finicky eater. She was always trying to get her daughter to eat more.

The woman's question brought to my mind the research of Leann Birch, professor of human development and family studies at Pennsylvania State University. Over the last 15 years, Birch has shown that kids are remarkably adept at adjusting their eating to meet their bodies' needs. One study, for example, demonstrated that children under the age of 5 spontaneously eat less when they are fed food that is rich in calories and eat more when the calorie content of the food is reduced.

"Left to their own devices," says Birch, "most kids do reasonably well in terms of adjusting how much and what they eat in response to the energy content of the diet. But parents can very easily put that off track by thinking that they need to take control of how much kids eat and really trying hard to control when, how much, and which foods kids eat." In fact, she says that parental control over meals is the best predictor of whether or not children will be able to adjust their food intake in experiments like the one just described.

What is scary is how easy it is to cross the line between being a parent who encourages a child's eating autonomy and being a controlling one. As examples of control, Birch lists encouraging children to eat only at mealtime rather than in response to hunger, or encouraging children to finish all the food given to them. She says people qualify as controlling if they believe that their job as a parent is not only to provide healthy food choices but to make sure that their children get enough of these foods.

The fact that children who have their eating decisions made for them do not learn self-control coincides with other research on the relationship between parenting style and children's development. The irony is that parents tend to be most controlling in areas where they themselves are highly invested. Parents who have trouble with their own eating tend to be most involved in their children's meals. They may be trying to do the best by their kids, but unfortunately their efforts backfire. "Parents who are out of control are producing kids who are out of control," says Birch, "by focusing them away from the internal hunger and satiety cues that would help them regulate how much and what they eat."

This seems to be particularly true when it comes to raising girls. In general, Birch has found that boys are better at regulating their intake than girls. Often girls who don't regulate well have mothers who are "restrained" eaters. That is, they count calories or follow strict diets in order to control their own weight. "We know that what's happening with slightly older girls," says Birch, "is that mothers are telling their daughters to diet and then telling them how to do it."

This sort of sabotage at home goes a long way toward explaining the craziness about dieting that is beginning to show up in preteen girls. More than half of middle-class 9- and 10-year-old girls in this country say they are dieting. Eating disorders are at an all time high, and 90 percent of the people affected are women. The unhealthy eating environment that surrounds many growing girls has only made them more vulnerable to cultural pressures to be thin.

The optimal environment, Birch says, is one in which parents provide healthy food choices but allow children to assume control over how much they eat. Parents can be assured that children will eat what and how much they need over the course of a day or two. This is true of the vast majority of children, whether they are overweight or not. Which is why, in the end, I told the woman on the airplane that my son knows better than I do how hungry he is. When he doesn't eat, I put the food away.

Get Moving

Six months before that flight, I was sitting in a lecture hall at one of the panel discussions on obesity that the Harvard School of Public Health in Boston periodically hosts. That day's symposium, called "Overweight America: Strategies for Change," was moderated by Steve Gortmaker, a senior lecturer on sociology at Harvard. Gortmaker has sandy, longish hair, and a breezy, comfortable manner. He can usually be counted on to bring cultural issues to the forefront of any health discussion, a knack that was on display that day during his opening remarks.

"Think of the food industry in the United States," he said. "To the extent that this multibillion-dollar industry is successful, is turning a profit, the population will consume more food. Think about television and the video, film, and video games industry. To the extent that this industry is successful in turning a profit, the entire population over time will become more and more inactive. These are fundamental forces I think are important to consider."

Such social issues have been at the heart of Gortmaker's research on obesity. One of his main contributions to the field during his career has been to focus attention on the effects of television viewing on weight. He has demonstrated a one-to-one relationship between the hours of television viewed daily and the prevalence of obesity. Although this could be interpreted as evidence that obesity causes people to spend more time watching TV, most studies have supported the opposite conclusion. It is television viewing that contributes to obesity.

Part of the reason for this association is that TV is such a sedentary activity. Watching TV slows down a person's metabolism to the point where they expend less energy than if they were doing nothing at all. Television, through its advertisements, can also increase the amount people eat while they're watching. And if eating in front of the TV is common, then it can become a conditioned stimulus to eat.

Children seem to be particularly vulnerable to these effects. One of Gortmaker's frequent collaborators is Bill Dietz at the CDC. Before moving to this agency in 1997, Dietz spent most of his career as a professor of pediatrics at Tufts University School of Medicine. Childhood obesity was his specialty, and thus, where Gortmaker has contributed the social perspective to the collaboration, Dietz has brought a focus on children.

About 35 percent of American children are now watching five or more hours of television a day compared to about 20 percent 25 years ago. Dietz and Gortmaker have found the same one-to-one relationship between TV and obesity in children that they found in adults. In a recent study, they looked at weight gain in a group of children over a four-year period and found that the odds of becoming obese were eight times higher for children watching more than five hours of television a day compared with those watching two or fewer hours a day.

"I think the notion that food is entertainment really begins in childhood," said Dietz during his remarks at the Harvard symposium that day. "And the food manufacturers have learned from the impact of television advertising on children to promote it to adults in the same fashion. If you watch the Saturday morning cereal ads or food ads, they're all about how much fun it is to eat it and how it'll make you feel great."

Perhaps the most intriguing thing to come out of the current focus on television is the realization that being more active and being less sedentary aren't necessarily the same thing. "We now know that sedentary activity, or inactivity, and activity have quite distinct and independent effects on the prevalence of obesity," Dietz continued. "They seem to operate independently and one is not the reciprocal of the other."

A good example of what Dietz means comes from a recent study by Leonard Epstein, a psychologist at the State University of New York at Buffalo. Epstein and his fellow researchers recruited obese kids, 8 to 12 years old, and divided them into three groups. One group was asked to increase the amount of time they spent exercising. If they did so, they received not only the praise of their parents, but a reward that the children and their parents had agreed upon in advance. Because Epstein's previous studies have shown that this sort of treatment works best when children also reinforce similar behavior in their parents, the adults also received rewards for being more active.

Epstein encouraged the second group of children to simply decrease the amount of time that they spent in sedentary activities. He rewarded them for not watching television, playing computer games, or talking on the phone—although not all sedentary activities were targeted. The kids could still listen to music or read for pleasure as well as do their homework. Finally, Epstein encouraged the third group of kids both to exercise more and to be less sedentary.

You would think that exercising would have a bigger effect on weight than not being sedentary. You might also assume that doing both would have the biggest effect of all. Yet on both counts you would be wrong. The kids in Epstein's study who experienced the largest drop in percentage overweight after a year were those who merely tried to be less sedentary.

Why would lounging around less be a better route to weight control than exercising more? Perhaps because when kids are denied sedentary activities they choose more active alternatives, Epstein says, whereas kids who exercise more can still be sedentary the rest of the time. Both at the beginning and the end of the study, Epstein asked the less sedentary kids what kinds of activities they preferred. Over the course of the year they showed the biggest boost in interest for high-intensity activities, which lends some support to this theory.

Epstein's results suggest that reducing access to television, computers, and other demons of sedentariness may combat the increasing level of obesity among children. But the fact that all of the kids in the study had enrolled willingly is also a hint that asking kids to cut down on their TV viewing won't necessarily have the same effect for all kids. As anyone with children understands all too well, helping kids develop more active lifestyles isn't as simple as clicking off the TV set. Not only are playgrounds and ball fields not readily available outside many kids' doors, but even when they are, children don't respond too cheerfully to having their TV privileges revoked.

Indeed Epstein seems to be mining a vein of truth when he suggests that the somewhat surprising results of his study may have to do with giving children choices and control over their lives. He points out that the kids who were asked to exercise more had to take time away from activities they would normally be doing. In contrast, the kids who were only expected to be less sedentary had the opportunity to choose what to do with that time. The mere fact that they were in control of that choice may have made them happier with whatever activity they decided to substitute. Why should they be any different from adults, after all?

An Ounce of Prevention

The fact is, we all respond best to choices and to a feeling of control over our lives. This is a lesson that applies not only to how we allocate our time each day but to the life-long struggle to achieve and maintain a healthy weight. To succeed in this struggle, we each need to tailor our approach to our own lives and our own bodies. Reducing the time we spend watching television and resisting the cultural pressures to diet are two important tools. There are many tools available, both now and in the coming years, to help people come to terms with their weight.

As research on weight continues to bombard us with new findings, one of the most important decisions that we will face is determining what constitutes a healthy body. Reasonable people still have widely divergent opinions on that issue. To some, excess fat is an overemphasized health statistic. Such was the thrust of a January 1, 1998, editorial in the *New England Journal of Medicine* by its editors, Jerome Kassirer and Marcia Angell. "Until we have better data about the risks of being overweight and the benefits and risks of trying to lose weight," they wrote, "we should remember that the cure for obesity may be worse than the condition."

That editorial raised the ire of those for whom obesity remains a deadly health scourge. In the months after its publication, former surgeon general C. Everett Koop and a host of other eminent parties publicly chastised the editors for trivializing the risks of excess weight. To those of us who are merely trying to sort out the best course for ourselves and our families, such conflicting messages can be exasperating. If the so-called experts can't agree on a basic issue like whether or not we should lose weight, who can we turn to for guidance?

In the midst of this confusion, however, there is one message on which nearly all the participants in the health debate agree: everyone's first priority should be preventing further weight gain. "No matter where you are in the population," says Bill Dietz, "even if you're overweight, the most important first step is to maintain your weight, not to gain weight further, because that's associated with a substantial increase in risk."

Some of the most interesting research indicating how large an effect prevention of weight gain can have on health comes from a group of rhesus monkeys in Barbara Hansen's lab at the University of Maryland School of Medicine. About a dozen years ago, Hansen put a group of rhesus monkeys on a weight-maintenance diet—one that bears some resemblance to the ritual many people practice daily.

"I like to refer to it as the bathroom scale model," Hansen told me over the phone from her Baltimore office. "If you get on the bathroom scale each day or at least once a week, and if you gain a little weight, you cut back your calories a little to get back to whatever you were. And if you lose a little weight, you add a few calories, and you just keep yourself stable. It's not a starvation diet. It's not an 800-calorie diet. It's not a 1200-calorie diet. It's just making sure you don't gain weight after you're an adult."

Since physical activity has consistently been associated with weight maintenance in people, I asked Hansen if she also had her monkeys on some sort of exercise program. She laughed. "For monkeys, like humans, exercise is not rewarding," she said. "Although there are a few humans out there who believe it is, they're crazy. And therefore the only way to make a monkey exercise is to do one of two things. Either electric shock them, and we don't do that kind of study anymore, or starve them and make them work for food. Well, that would ruin the experiment. So the monkeys are just what you would call normally active. They're not hyperactive. There just isn't any way to force them to exercise."

Again, this is a level of activity that average people could envision themselves doing, particularly if the health benefits were as remarkable as those Hansen saw in her monkeys. "By preventing them from gaining weight, we totally prevented the development of type II diabetes," said Hansen. "Whereas the control group, at least half of them are diabetic or showing signs of becoming diabetic." Left to eat as they wished, the monkeys in the control group have spontaneously gained weight as they have aged.

Can people who hold their weight constant as they grow older expect the same sort of health benefit? Hansen says, "Everything we have discovered in the monkeys has proven also to be true in humans, if it's been looked for. Everything. They have the same insulin as in humans. It's identical in structure. They develop the same disease. Type II diabetes is obesity associated, just like human disease."

Based on studies like Hansen's, as well as a wealth of research on type II diabetes in people, the National Institutes of Health has launched a large-scale trial in which they will try to stop, or at least slow, weight gain to see if they can prevent the development of type II diabetes. Begun in 1996, the trial is proceeding at 25 medical sites across the United States. Its earliest results are at least five years away.

Many researchers suspect that people will have an easier time preventing weight gain than maintaining a loss, but that has yet to be proven. Despite the evidence of prevention's health benefits, researchers have no track record of success in keeping people from gaining weight. And no one believes it is going to be easy. After all, these are people, not monkeys, and even the monkeys in Hansen's study weren't entirely satisfied with their weight-maintenance diet. On the rare occasions when they were allowed to eat extra—when a technician accidentally gave them too much food, for example—they ate every speck of it. The people in the trial will have the same urges, yet there will be no caretaker restricting their access to more calories.

What this trial does have going for it is its open-eyed approach. It fully embraces what researchers have learned so far about the biological underpinnings of weight. Instead of doing battle with our body's natural defenses, it attempts to work with them. Its goal of prevention, while still untested, is a reasonable long-term strategy for people of all weight classes. And unlike many previous trials which have seen weight as the primary health threat, this trial focuses on the risk factors of illness.

These are all signs that America's nationwide journey toward weight control has taken a positive and more informed turn. For so many years we have been groping in the dark for solutions to weight problems. People who struggle with their weight as well as those who study it have repeatedly been seduced and then betrayed by such solutions. The result has been immeasurable frustration. Now scientific research on weight is taking us into an entirely new terrain. In the ongoing effort to both understand our bodies and gain some control of them, there is reason to hope that the frustration is nearing an end.

Acknowledgments

Writing a book is never easy, but my task was made considerably easier by the kindness and assistance of a number of people. During the early stages of researching this book, I benefitted from the hospitality of the men and women who make up the Boston Obesity/Nutrition Center's Epidemiology Working Group. They welcomed me at their biweekly meetings on a range of ongoing research topics, and though I rarely participated in the discussions, I drew immeasurable insight from them.

Dozens of other scientists spent time explaining their particular type of obesity research to me and sharing their views of the history and progress of this field. For memorably thoughtful and enlightening conversations, I owe special thanks to Arthur Frank, Barbara Hansen, Xavier Pi-Sunyer, David West, and Art Campfield. Ditto for size activist Lynn McAfee, who in some ways saw the scientists more clearly than they saw themselves.

As this book progressed from proposal to draft to final product, it also benefitted from the scrutiny of many people. Some of the earliest readers were friends whose questions and criticisms improved the book immeasurably: George Pace, Angelia Pippin, Anjali Sastry, and the members of my book group, Michelle Kaczynski, Mary Austin Dowd, Melinda Harrison, Sarah Bassett, and Kathy Rogers. Early on, Clay Shirky also expressed the hope that the book would be "relevant," and his wish continuously lurked in the back of my mind.

Victor McElheny and the ever-changing roster of people at the Knight Science Journalism Fellowships at MIT gave me dose after dose of encouragement. They also served as a constant reminder to keep my standards high.

I want to thank Elizabeth Knoll for acquiring the book and for many thought-provoking discussions during its early stages. My editor, Holly Hodder, worked tirelessly to make the book as clear and engaging as it could be. Regula Noetzli has been my agent since I began writing books. In that time she has earned my undying gratitude for her mince-no-words approach to the business and her inherent good sense.

Last, and most important, I would like to convey my heartfelt thanks to the members of my family, who both inspired this book and supported me through the most difficult parts of writing it. My mother, Virginia, witnessed only the early stages of the book, but her memory sat on my shoulder whenever I worked. My sister Valorie gave me her unfailing honesty about a topic that has been fundamental in her life. My son Maceo taught me to see the world through an entirely new set of eyes. My dearest Conrad showered me with ideas, advice, enthusiasm, and his unshakable belief in my abilities. For him, I am most grateful of all.

Sources

INTRODUCTION
Page
1   **In 1993 the American Association for the Advancement of Science sponsored . . .** "Human Obesity: Current Status of Scientific and Clinical Progress," February 12–13, 1993, two-day seminar at AAAS'93, Boston. Organized by David Allison and F. Xavier Pi-Sunyer.

3   **And late the following year, one of those seeds produced . . .** Yiying Zhang, Ricardo Proenca, Margherita Maffei, Marisa Barone, Lori Leopold and Jeffrey Friedman, "Positional cloning of the mouse *obese* gene and its human homologue," *Nature*, December 1, 1994, vol. 372, pp. 425–432.

5   **A quarter of Americans are obese . . .** Robert Kuczmarski et al., "Increasing prevalence of overweight among U.S. adults: National Health and Nutrition Examination Surveys, 1960 to 1991," *Journal of the American Medical Association*, July 20, 1994, vol. 272, no. 3, pp. 205–211.

5   **Recently John Foreyt . . .** J. Foreyt and K. Goodrick, "The ultimate triumph of obesity," *Lancet*, July 15, 1995, vol. 346, no. 8968, pp. 134–135.

5   **While the rates in most other westernized nations . . .** Gary Taubes, "Weight increases worldwide?" *Science*, May 29, 1998, vol. 280, p. 1368.

8   **Maybe just moderate exercise . . .** Russell R. Pate et al., "Physical activity and public health: A recommendation from the Centers for Disease Control and Prevention and the American College of Sports Medicine," *Journal of the American Medical Association*, February 1, 1995, vol. 273, no. 5, pp. 402–407.

9   **. . . references to the idea that obesity is a disease— a chronic illness . . .** B. T. Burton, W. R. Foster, J. Hirsch, and T. B. Van Itallie, "Health implications of obesity: An NIH Consensus Development Conference," *International Journal of Obesity*, 1985, vol. 9, pp. 155–170.

9   **. . . a public health threat that costs our nation . . .** Anne M. Wolf and Graham A. Colditz, "Current estimates of the economic cost of obesity in the United States," *Obesity Research*, March 1998, vol. 6, no. 2, pp. 97–106.

9   **Over the next decade we will be seeing . . .** Interview with Leo Lutwak, a medical officer with the Center for Drug Evaluation, Food and Drug Administration, February 10, 1997.

10   **For now the mantra among many obesity specialists is prevention . . .** World Health Organization, *Obesity: Preventing and Managing the Global Epidemic* (World Health Organization, 1998).

One
ALL IN THE FAMILY

13 **John Rossi had worked . . .** Interview with Barbara Lawless, April 28, 1997. Kathleen Sullivan, "Fired for being fat, he wins $1 million," *San Francisco Examiner*, September 7, 1995, p. A8.

14 **Under the same law, a Santa Cruz woman . . .** *Cassista v. Community Foods Inc.*, September 2, 1993. Ellen Moskowitz, "In the courts: Am I disabled?" *Hastings Center Report*, May-June 1994. Interview with Maureen Arrigo-Ward, California Western School of Law, April 21, 1997.

14 **And if that were truly the case, it would have been very much in agreement . . .** EEOC Compliance Manual, vol. 2, sec. 902. Interview with Susan Adams, attorney advisor, Office of Legal Counsel, EEOC, April 16, 1997.

15 **Lynette Labinger was loath to make the same mistake . . .** Interview with Lynette Labinger, April 22, 1997. *Bonnie Cook v. State of Rhode Island*, Department of Mental Health, Retardation and Hospitals, November 22, 1993.

16 **"Nature does not permit body weight to fluctuate" . . .** Arthur Frank, "Futility and avoidance: Medical professionals in the treatment of obesity," *Journal of the American Medical Association*, April 28, 1993, vol. 269, no. 16, pp. 2132–2133.

18 **. . . the 80 percent figure is at the high end . . .** Claude Bouchard and Louis Perusse, "Genetics of obesity," *Annual Review of Nutrition*, 1993, vol. 13, pp. 337–354.

19   **For over 20 years, families of French descent** . . .
Interview with Claude Bouchard, February 3, 1995.

20   **Paul-André Sauvageau, a retired civil engineer** . . .
Interview with Sauvageau, February 9, 1995.

21   **But studies during the mid-1980s of identical twins** . . .
A. J. Stunkard, T. T. Foch, and Z. Hrubec, "A twin study
of human obesity," *Journal of the American Medical
Association*, 1986, vol. 256, pp. 51–54. A. J. Stunkard, J.
R. Harris, N. L. Pederson, and G. E. McClearn, "The
body mass index of twins who have been reared apart,"
New England Journal of Medicine, 1990, vol. 322,
pp. 1483–1487.

23   **Bouchard and his colleagues have amassed information on** . . . Bouchard and Perusse, 1993. C. Bouchard
and F. E. Johnston (Eds.), *Fat Distribution During
Growth and Later Health Outcomes* (Alan Liss, 1988).

25   **Jose Caro, an obesity specialist at Lilly Research
Labs** . . . Interview with Caro, August 17, 1995.

26   **Charles Rotimi, an obesity researcher at the Loyola
University Medical Center** . . . Charles N. Rotimi et al.,
"Distribution of anthropometric variables and the
prevalence of obesity in populations of West African
origin: International Collaborative Study on
Hypertension in Blacks," *Obesity Research*, September
2, 1995, vol. 3, suppl. 2, pp. 95s–105s. Interview with
Rotimi, December 15, 1997.

28   **"Some people have the good genes"** . . . D. B. West,
B. York, J. Waguespack, J. Goudey-Lefevre, and A. R.
Price, "Genetics of dietary obesity in AKR/J x SWR/J
mice: Segregation of the trait and identification of a
linked locus on chromosome 4, *Mammalian Genome*,

1994, vol. 5, pp. 546–552. Interview with David West, February 5, 1997.

32   **"You've got to have an explanation"** . . . Interview with Richard Surwit, July 31, 1997.

33   **A group of researchers at Rockefeller University** . . . Interview with David West, February 5, 1997.

33   **Recently Bouchard and his colleagues used their extensive list** . . . Yvon C. Chagnon et al., "Suggestive linkages between markers on human 1p32–p22 and body fat and insulin levels in the Quebec Family Study," *Obesity Research*, March 1997, vol. 5, no. 2, pp. 115–119.

34   **Over the last ten years Bouchard and his collaborators** . . . Bouchard and Perusse, 1993.

35   **Another distinct major gene affects resting metabolic rate** . . . Treva Rice, Angelo Tremblay, Olivier Deriaz, Louis Perusse, D. C. Rao, and Claude Bouchard, "A major gene for resting metabolic rate unassociated with body composition: Results from the Quebec Family Study," *Obesity Research*, September 1996, vol. 4, no. 5, pp. 441–449.

36   **Nearly half of Americans consider themselves overweight** . . . John Horm and Kay Anderson, "Who in America is trying to lose weight?" *Annals of Internal Medicine*, October 1, 1993, vol. 119, no. 7 (part 2), pp. 672–676.

Two
OF MICE AND MEN

37   **One day during the summer** . . . Ann Ingalls, Margaret Dickie, and G. D. Snell, "Obese, a new mutation in the house mouse," *Journal of Heredity*, 1950, vol. 41, no. 12, pp. 317–318.

37   **At that time, Bar Harbor** . . . *Bar Harbor Times*, 1996 Bicentennial Souvenir Edition, pp.11–14.

38   **The Jackson Laboratory is an institution** . . . Jean Holstein, *The First Fifty Years at the Jackson Laboratory* (Jackson Laboratory, 1979), pp. 1–36.

38   **. . . voluntarily cutting their salaries by two-thirds** . . . Ibid., pp. 18–21.

39   **. . . had routinely been treated with creosote and kerosene** . . . Ibid., p. 39.

40   **There was only one other genetically fat mouse** . . . C. H. Danforth, "Hereditary adiposity in mice," *Journal of Heredity*, 1927, vol. 18, pp. 153–162.

40   **. . . Dickie danced into the lab director's office** . . . Interview with Priscilla (Skippy) Lane, August 26, 1996.

41   **The plump mouse had made the cover** . . . *Journal of Heredity*, 1950, vol. 41, no. 12.

41   **The *ob* mouse came into a world** . . . Hillel Schwartz, *Never Satisfied: A Cultural History of Diets, Fantasies and Fat* (Doubleday, 1986), p. 204.

41   **. . . Milwaukee housewife Esther Manz had read an article** . . . Roberta Pollack Seid, *Never Too Thin: Why Women Are at War with Their Bodies* (Prentice Hall, 1989), p. 107.

41   **. . . those who lost weight were literally crowned as royalty** . . . "Esther Manz" (obituary), *The Economist*, March 16, 1996, p. 88.

41   **In the prosperous decade following the war** . . . Seid, p. 128.

42   **. . . declared obesity to be the nation's number one nutrition problem** . . . "Obesity is now no. 1 U.S. nutritional problem," *Science News Letter*, December 27, 1952, vol. 62, p. 408.

42   **One of the most popular was** . . . Schwartz,
      pp. 198–199. Seid, pp. 105–106.

43   **"The old tradition that obese people are psychiatri-
      cally ill"** . . . Interview with Xavier Pi-Sunyer,
      September 4, 1996.

45   **That was the thinking of nutritionist Jean Mayer** . . .
      Holstein, pp. 154–155.

45   **"He would complain all the time"** . . . Interview with
      Douglas Coleman, January 12, 1995.

48   **. . . the 1970s saw many obesity researchers turning
      their attention** . . . George Bray, "Eat slowly—From
      laboratory to clinic: Behavioral control of eating,"
      Obesity Research, July 1996, vol. 4, no. 4, pp. 397–400.

49   **Stuart took a handful of overweight patients** . . .
      Richard B. Stuart, "Behavioral control of overeating,"
      Behaviour Research and Therapy, 1967, vol. 5, pp. 357–365.

50   **In the hands of thoughtful practitioners** . . . Albert
      Stunkard, "Diet, exercise and behavior therapy: A cau-
      tionary tale," *Obesity Research*, May 1996, vol. 4, no. 3,
      pp. 293–294.

51   **The same year, 47 percent of Americans** . . .
      Schwartz, p. 255.

51   **The 1970s were also a historic decade for molecular
      biology** . . . Jerry Bishop and Michael Waldholz,
      Genome (Simon and Schuster, 1990), pp. 49–102.

53   **Jeffrey Friedman was one such biologist** . . .
      Interview with Friedman, January 12, 1995.

55   **This work narrowed the location of the gene** . . .
      Yiying Zhang, Ricardo Proenca, Margherita Maffei,
      Marisa Barone, Lori Leopold, and Jeffrey Friedman,
      "Positional cloning of the mouse *obese* gene and its
      human homologue," *Nature*, December 1, 1994, vol. 372,

pp. 425–432. Interview with Yiying Zhang, January 12, 1995.

57   **One day, RNA for one of the genes they were testing showed up only in fat . . .** Friedman, lecture at Harvard Medical School, May 8, 1996.

59   **In an informal test during the weeks following the gene discovery . . .** Friedman, lecture at Massachusetts Institute of Technology, March 27, 1995.

60   **. . . most obese people had too much leptin floating around their bodies . . .** Margherita Maffei et al., "Leptin levels in human and rodent: Measurement of plasma leptin and *ob* RNA in obese and weight-reduced subjects," *Nature Medicine*, November 1995, vol. 1, no. 11, pp. 1155–1161.

60   **On the day the *Nature* paper came out, Friedman appeared live . . .** Transcript of CNN Live Report, December 1, 1994.

62   **At a gathering of his fellow biologists . . .** Friedman, lecture at MIT.

Three
NO, THEY CAN'T TAKE
THAT AWAY FROM ME

65   **On a bright Saturday morning . . .** Taping session at Speer Communications Studio, Nashville, Tennessee, November 1, 1997.

66   **"You dress for it. You put on" . . .** Rob Scobey, item in the online newsletter *Weigh Down Digest*, October 6, 1997, http://wdworkshop.com.

66   **Shamblin's solution to this problem is for people . . .** Gwen Shamblin, *The Weigh Down Diet* (Doubleday, 1997), p. 6.

66   **Since the 1950s, Christian-based diets have made up . . .** R. Marie Griffith, "The promised land of weight loss: Law and gospel in Christian dieting," *The Christian Century*, May 7, 1997, pp. 448–454. Hillel Schwartz, *Never Satisfied: A Cultural History of Diets, Fantasies and Fat* (Doubleday, 1986), pp. 307–310. Roberta Pollack Seid, *Never Too Thin: Why Women Are at War with Their Bodies* (Prentice Hall, 1989), p. 168.

67   **. . . from Catherine of Siena, who ate only herbs, to Eva Fleigen . . .** Joan Jacobs Brumberg, *Fasting Girls: The History of Anorexia Nervosa* (Plume, 1989), pp. 41–60.

68   **A so-called "normal" eater as a girl . . .** Shamblin, *The Weigh Down Diet*, pp. 13–20.

71   **"Diets do not work because they are basically" . . .** Ibid., pp. 29, 83.

72   **Furthermore, while Shamblin may have her mind . . .** *Weigh Down Digest*, October 6, 1997.

72   **Such has been the fate of many diet books . . .** Barry Sears, with Bill Lawren, *Enter The Zone* (Harper Collins, 1995). Robert C. Atkins, *Dr. Atkins' New Diet Revolution* (Avon Books, 1992).

73   **One popular regime that recently . . .** Monique P. Yazigi, "Melt pounds with cabbage soup, a diet from nowhere says," *The New York Times*, March 20, 1996, p. C3.

73   **. . . the subtraction stew that was served . . .** Norton Juster, *The Phantom Tollbooth* (Epstein & Carroll; distributed by Random House, 1961) p. 185.

73   **A friend from Holland recently told me about her encounter . . .** Conversation with Marjo van der Meulen, February 22, 1997.

74   **High-protein diets like The Zone operate on a similar principle . . .** Bonnie Liebman, "Where's the evidence,"

Nutrition Action Healthletter, April 1997, p. 11. Barry Sears, "Defending The Zone," *Nutrition Action Healthletter*, April 1997, p. 10. Questioning 40/30/30, a joint statement put out by the American College of Sports Medicine, the American Dietetic Association, the Women's Sports Foundation, and the Cooper Institute for Aerobics Research.

75   **One-fourth of all Americans are insulin resistant . . .** Molly O'Neill, "So it may be true after all: Eating pasta makes you fat," *The New York Times*, February 8, 1995, p. A1.

75   **Chris Rosenbloom, a nutritionist at Georgia State University in Atlanta . . .** Sheryl Julian, "This diet is great," *Boston Globe*, February 18, 1998, p. C1.

77   **In 1995 three scientists from Rockefeller University . . .** Rudolph Leibel, Michael Rosenbaum, and Jules Hirsch, "Changes in energy expenditure resulting from altered body weight," *New England Journal of Medicine*, March 9, 1995, vol. 332, no. 10, pp. 621–628.

77   **The idea that the body has a set weight that it defends . . .** George Bray, "Static theories in a dynamic world: A glucodynamic theory of food intake," *Obesity Research*, September 1996, vol. 4, no. 5, pp. 489–492.

80   **These questions were addressed in an editorial . . .** William Ira Bennett, "Beyond overeating," *New England Journal of Medicine*, March 9, 1995, vol. 332, no. 10, pp. 673–674.

81   **As a result, our bodies have developed a variety of defenses . . .** Jeffrey Friedman, "The alphabet of weight control," *Nature*, January 9, 1997, vol. 385, pp. 119–120.

81   **While many researchers initially called leptin a "satiety signal" . . .** Timothy Rink, "In search of a satiety

factor," *Nature*, December 1, 1994, vol. 372, pp. 406–407. Jeffrey Flier, remarks during a lecture at Harvard Medical School, September 16, 1996.

81 **. . . is probably what the leptin molecule evolved to do . . .** Rexford S. Ahima, Daniel Prabakaran, Christos Mantzoros, Daqing Qu, Bradford Lowell, Eleftheria Maratos-Flier, and Jeffrey S. Flier, "Role of leptin in the neuroendocrine response to fasting," *Nature*, July 18, 1996, vol. 382, pp. 250–252.

82 **Leptin levels also appear to be linked to a delay . . .** V. Matkovic et al., "Leptin is inversely related to age at menarche in human females," *Journal of Clinical Endocrinology and Metabolism*, October 1997, vol. 82, no. 10, pp. 3239–3245. Jeffrey Flier, lecture at Harvard Medical School, September 16, 1996.

82 **A drop in leptin boosts the levels of . . .** Friedman, "The alphabet of weight control," pp. 119–120.

82 **Sarah Leibowitz, a neurobiologist at Rockefeller University, has spent . . .** Interview with Leibowitz, April 26, 1996.

82 **According to Leibowitz, NPY is particularly adept at . . .** M. Jhanwar-Uniyal, B. Beck, Y. S. Jhanwar, C. Burlet, and S. F. Leibowitz, "Neuropeptide Y projection from arcuate nucleus to parvocellular division of the paraventricular nucleus: Specific relation to the ingestion of carbohydrate," *Brain Research*, 1993, vol. 631, p. 97.

83 **Researchers studying the effects of artificial sweeteners . . .** J. H. Lavin, S. J. French, and N. W. Read, "The effect of sucrose- and aspartame-sweetened drinks on energy intake, hunger and food choice of female, moderately restrained eaters," *International Journal of Obesity*, January 1997, vol. 21, no. 1, pp. 37–42.

84   **However, fat seems to be less clearly regulated than . . .**
      Andrew Prentice (Ed), "Obesity: Are all calories equal?"
      International Journal of Obesity, November 1995, vol. 19,
      suppl. 5, pp. S1–S43. Arne Astrup et al., "Obesity as an
      adaptation to a high-fat diet: Evidence from a cross-
      sectional study," *American Journal of Clinical Nutrition*,
      February 1994, vol. 59, no. 2, pp. 350–355.

85   **Olestra was first discovered in the late 1960s . . .**
      Wendy Jacques, spokesperson for Procter and Gamble,
      May 1996. Myra Karstadt, lecture at Harvard School of
      Public Health, April 5, 1996.

87   **Researchers at Pennsylvania State University, in col-
      laboration . . .** D. L. Miller, V. A. Hammer, J. C. Peters,
      and B. J. Rolls, "Effects of substituting fat-free (olestra)
      potato chips on 24-hour fat and energy intake," *Obesity
      Research*, October 3, 1995, vol. 3, suppl. 3, p. 327s.

88   **The classic study proving this connection was
      done . . .** Ancel Keys, J. Brozek, A. Henschel, O.
      Michelson, and H. Longhurst, *Biology of Human
      Starvation* (University of Minnesota Press, 1950).

89   **Keys's study is one of many that University of
      Toronto psychologist . . .** Janet Polivy and C. Peter
      Herman, *Breaking the Diet Habit: The Natural Weight
      Alternative* (Basic Books, 1983), p. 198.

89   **. . . believes people rarely get fat by going on binges
      but instead . . .** J. Polivy and C. P. Herman, "Dieting
      and bingeing: A causal analysis," *American Journal of
      Public Health*, 1985, vol. 40, pp. 193–201.

91   **Gwen Shamblin refers to such people as having . . .**
      Taping session at Speer Communications Studio, 1997.

91   **Such an obsession affects Kay . . .** Conversations and
      correspondence with participant in Weigh Down
      Workshop, April 1997–June 1998.

93   **They are a journey back to the days** . . . L. L. Birch, "Children's food intake: A developmental perspective," *Obesity Research*, October 3, 1995, vol. 3, suppl. 3, p. 307s.

94   **"Giving up dieting, especially for fat women, is not"** . . . Andria Siegler, "Grieving the lost dreams of thinness." In Catrina Brown and Karin Jasper (Eds.), *Consuming Passions: Feminist Approaches to Weight Preoccupation and Eating Disorders* (Second Story Press, 1993), p. 153.

95   **"It's a process that doesn't take place overnight"** . . . Cheri Erdman, lecture at NAAFA meeting, July 10, 1996.

96   **Experience with Beyond Dieting has shown** . . . Donna Ciliska, "Beyond Dieting," in *Consuming Passions*, pp. 382–389.

98   **"The motivation to be thin is not vanity—it is natural"** . . . Shamblin, *The Weigh Down Diet*, p. 5.

Four
THE SUCCESSFUL LOSER

101   **To Dominguez, this is all a familiar routine** . . . Interview with Marisol Dominguez, September 4, 1996.

101   **"Okay, now let's go through the test again"** . . . Interview with Albert Kovera, September 4, 1996.

104   **During a conversation that obesity researcher James Hill** . . . Interview with Hill, September 10, 1996.

104   **This was the conclusion drawn by** . . . NIH Technology Assessment Conference Panel, "Methods for voluntary weight loss and control: Technology Assessment Conference statement," *Annals of Internal Medicine*, 1993, vol. 119, pp. 764–770.

105   **Instead, 95 percent of men and 87 percent of**

women . . . Institute of Medicine, *Weighing the Options: Criteria for Evaluating Weight-Management Programs* (National Academy Press, 1995), p. 27.

105 **A somewhat unscientific survey may provide . . .** "Rating the diets," *Consumer Reports*, June 1993, pp. 353–357.

105 **They contacted the Sandoz Corporation . . .** Hill, September 10, 1996.

107 **Hill has just the tool to make that happen . . .** Interview with Teresa Sharp, September 10, 1996.

108 **. . . some conclusions can be drawn . . .** Hill, September 10, 1996.

110 **The same conclusions Hill and Wing are drawing . . .** Interview with Barbara Hansen, August 28, 1996.

112 **They increased their physical activity enormously . . .** M. L. Klem, R. R. Wing, M. T. McGuire, H. M. Seagle, and J. O. Hill, "A descriptive study of individuals successful at long-term maintenance of substantial weight loss," *American Journal of Clinical Nutrition*, August 1997, vol. 66, no. 2, pp. 239–246.

112 **There are several ways exercise may help . . .** "Proceedings of a satellite symposium of the 7th International Congress on Obesity on exercise and obesity: Morphological, metabolic and clinical implications," *International Journal of Obesity*, October 1995, vol. 19, suppl. 4, pp. s1–s128.

112 **. . . while you are exercising, your body burns more calories . . .** K. R. Segal, "Exercise and thermogenesis in obesity," *International Journal of Obesity*, October 1995, vol. 19, suppl. 4, pp. s80–s87.

112 **. . . your overall metabolism is cranked up for some time after . . .** Angelo Tremblay and Benjamin Buemann, "Exercise-training, macronutrient balance

and body weight control" (review), *International Journal of Obesity*, 1995, vol. 19, pp. 79–86.

113 **How long enhanced metabolism continues depends . . .** James O. Hill and John C. Peters, "Exercise and macronutrient balance," *International Journal of Obesity*, October 1995, vol. 19, suppl. 4, pp. s88–s92.

113 **Of all the weight-loss techniques that have been tried . . .** C. M. Grilo, K. D. Brownell, and A. J. Stunkard, "The metabolic and psychological importance of exercise in weight control." In A. J. Stunkard and T. A. Wadden (Eds.), *Obesity: Theory and Therapy* (Raven Press, 1993), pp. 253–274.

114 **Recently John Foreyt's lab, at the Baylor College of Medicine . . .** M. L. Skender, G. K. Goodrick, D. J. Del Junco, R. S. Reeves, L. Darnell, A. M. Gotto, and J. P. Foreyt, "Comparison of 2-year weight loss trends in behavioral treatments of obesity: Diet, exercise and combination interventions," *Journal of the American Dietetic Association*, April 1996, vol. 96, no. 4, pp. 342–346.

114 **Kelly Brownell, a psychologist and director of the Yale . . .** Kelly D. Brownell, "Exercise and obesity treatment: psychological aspects," *International Journal of Obesity*, October 1995, vol. 19, suppl. 4, pp. s122–s125.

115 **Most dieters know that it is much easier to cut calories by eating fewer . . .** Per Bjorntorp, "Evolution of the understanding of the role of exercise in obesity and its complications," *International Journal of Obesity*, October 1995, vol. 19, suppl. 4, pp. s1–s4.

115 **For example, in one study in which obese people . . .** John P. Foreyt, Robert L. Brunner, G. Ken Goodrick, Sachiko T. St. Jeor, and Grant Miller, "Psychological correlates of reported physical activity in normal-weight

and obese adults: The Reno diet-heart study," *International Journal of Obesity*, October 1995, vol. 19, suppl. 4, pp. s69–s72.

117 **In a survey of over 4,000 readers of *Runner's World* magazine . . .** K. D. Brownell, J. Rodin, and J. H. Wilmore, "Eat, drink and be worried?" *Runner's World*, August 1988, pp. 28–34.

117 **. . . exercise, despite all the weight benefits mentioned . . .** J. H. Wilmore, "Variations in physical activity habits and body composition," *International Journal of Obesity*, 1995, vol. 19, suppl. 4, pp. s107–s112.

118 **"Quite frankly, I think fitness is more important" . . .** Interview with Steven Blair, June 23, 1997.

118 **The invitation prompted him to look specifically . . .** Carolyn E. Barlow, Harold W. Kohl, Larry W. Gibbons, and Steven N. Blair, "Physical fitness, mortality and obesity," *International Journal of Obesity*, 1995, vol. 19, suppl. 4, pp. s41–s44.

121 **At conferences, scientists still worry out loud that people . . .** Interview with Glenn Gaesser, May 29, 1997.

121 **The summary of the research on people of all shapes, sizes . . .** Russell R. Pate et al., "Physical activity and public health: A recommendation from the Centers for Disease Control and Prevention and the American College of Sports Medicine," *Journal of the American Medical Association*, February 1, 1995, vol. 273, no. 5, pp. 402–407.

121 **Regular physical activity can improve insulin sensitivity . . .** V. A. Koivisto, H. Yki-Jarvinen, and R. A. DeFronzo, "Physical training and insulin sensitivity," *Diabetes and Metabolism Reviews*, 1986, vol. 1, pp. 445–481.

121   **. . . and blood pressure. . . .** Robert S. Schwartz and Victor A. Hirth, "The effects of endurance and resistance training on blood pressure," *International Journal of Obesity*, October 1995, vol. 19, suppl. 4, pp. s52–s57.

121   **It can increase the level of . . .** W. L. Haskell, "The influence of exercise training on plasma lipids and lipoproteins in health and disease," *Acta Medica Scandinavica*, 1986, vol. 711 (suppl.), pp. 25–37.

121   **One of the many ways exercise provides these benefits . . .** E. R. Nadel, "Circulatory and thermal regulations during exercise," *Federation Proceedings*, April 1980, vol. 39, no. 5, pp. 1491–1497.

121   **It takes only a single, intense exercise session to boost the total volume . . .** C. M. Gillen, R. Lee, G. W. Mack, C. M. Tomaselli, T. Nishiyaso, and E. R. Nadel, "Plasma volume expansion in humans after a single intense exercise protocol," *Journal of Applied Physiology*, November 1991, vol. 71, no. 5, pp. 1914–1920.

122   **. . . our hearts not only beat faster but pump more blood . . .** C. M. Gillen, T. Nishiyasu, G. Langhans, C. Weseman, G. W. Mack, and E. R. Nadel, "Cardiovascular and renal function during exercise-induced blood volume expansion in men," *Journal of Applied Physiology*, June 1994, vol. 76, no. 6, pp. 2602–2610.

122   **The resting heart rates of athletes are about . . .** B. Desvaux, P. Abraham, D. Colin, G. Leftheriotis, and J. L. Saumet, "Ankle to arm index following maximal exercise in normal subjects and athletes," *Medicine and Science in Sports and Exercise*, July 1996, vol. 28, no. 7, pp. 836–839.

122 **. . . physically fit people get fewer colds and other respiratory . . .** D. C. Nieman, "Physical activity, fitness, and infection." In C. Bouchard, R. J. Shephard, T. Stephens (Eds.), *Physical Activity, Fitness, and Health* (Human Kinetics Publishers; 1994), pp. 796–813.

123 **On a sunny July day in 1996, Al Gore and his wife . . .** Marion Burros, "Federal report promotes common-place exercise," *The New York Times*, July 12, 1996, p. A12.

123 **. . . 54 percent of adults fall short of the goal of 30 minutes . . .** U.S. Department of Health and Human Services, *Healthy People 2000: National Health Promotion and Disease Prevention Objectives*, DHHS Publication No. 91–50212 (Government Printing Office, 1991).

124 **The least sedentary adults are in the West . . .** "State surveys find few adults exercise enough," *The New York Times*, August 10, 1996, p. 12.

124 **One of the reasons many people shy away from exercise . . .** Committee to Develop Criteria for Evaluating the Outcomes of Approaches to Prevent and Treat Obesity, Paul R. Thomas (Ed.), Institute of Medicine, *Weighing the Options: Criteria for Evaluating Weight-Management Programs* (National Academy Press, 1995), p. 113.

124 **And despite what might be referred to as the Oprah Winfrey excuse . . .** Rena R. Wing, Robert W. Jeffery, Nocolaas Pronk, and Wendy L. Hellerstedt, "Effects of a personal trainer and financial incentives on exercise adherence in overweight women in a behavioral weight loss program," *Obesity Research*, September 1996, vol. 4, no. 5, pp. 457–462.

125 **It has been estimated that as many as 250,000 deaths per year** . . . R. A. Hahn, S. M. Teutsch, R. B. Rothenberg, and J. S. Marks, "Excess deaths from nine chronic diseases in the United States," *Journal of the American Medical Association*, 1986, vol. 264, pp. 2654–2659. J. M. McGinnis and W. H. Foege, "Actual causes of death in the United States," *Journal of the American Medical Association*, 1993, vol. 270, pp. 2207–2212.

125 **The evidence was laid out most convincingly** . . . Russell R. Pate et al., "Physical activity and public health: A recommendation from the Centers for Disease Control and Prevention and the American College of Sports Medicine," *Journal of the American Medical Association*, February 1, 1995, vol. 273, no. 5, pp. 402–407.

126 **The best argument that moderate activity provides** . . . S. N. Blair et al., "Changes in physical fitness and all-cause mortality. A prospective study of healthy and unhealthy men," *Journal of the American Medical Association*, April 12, 1995, vol. 273, pp. 1093–1098. R. S. Paffenbarger, Jr., et al., "Physical activity, all-cause mortality, and longevity of college alumni," *New England Journal of Medicine*, March 6, 1986, vol. 314, no. 10, pp. 605–613.

126 **One such study is known as the Multiple** . . . A. S. Leon et al., "Leisure-time physical activity levels and risk of coronary heart disease and death: The Multiple Risk Factor Intervention Trial," *Journal of the American Medical Association*, November 1987, vol. 258, no. 17, pp. 2388–2395. A. S. Leon et al., "Leisure-time physical activity and the 16-year risks of mortality from coronary heart disease and all-causes in the Multiple Risk

Factor Intervention Trial (MRFIT)," *International Journal of Sports Medicine*, July 1997, vol. 18, suppl. 3, pp. s208–s215.

126 **For example, John Duncan, an exercise physiologist . . .** J. J. Duncan, J. E. Farr, S. J. Upton, R. D. Hagan, M. E. Oglesby, and S. N. Blair, "The effects of aerobic exercise on plasma catecholamines and blood pressure in patients with mild essential hypertension," *Journal of the American Medical Association*, 1985, vol. 254, pp. 2609–2613.

127 **Critics like Paul Williams, an exercise researcher . . .** Marcia Barinaga, "How much pain for cardiac gain," *Science*, May 30, 1997, vol. 276, pp. 1324–1327.

128 **What's more, researchers like Abby King . . .** A. C. King, C. B. Taylor, and W. L. Haskell, "Effects of differing intensities and formats of 12 months of exercise training on psychological outcomes in older adults," *Health Psychology*, 1993, vol. 12, pp. 292–300. A. C. King et al., "Influence of regular aerobic exercise on psychological health," *Health Psychology*, 1989, vol. 8, pp. 305–324.

128 **The most direct evidence that piecemeal exercise "counts" . . .** R. F. DeBusk, U. Stenestrand, M. Sheehan, and W. W. L. Haskell, "Training effects of long versus short bouts of exercise in healthy subjects," *American Journal of Cardiology*, 1990, vol. 65, pp. 1010–1013.

129 **In addition, Rena Wing's group has found . . .** J. M. Jakicic, Rena Wing, B. A. Butler, and R. J. Robertson, "Prescribing exercise in multiple short bouts versus one continuous bout: Effects on adherence, cardiorespiratory fitness, and weight loss in overweight women,"

International Journal of Obesity, December 1995, vol. 19, no. 12, pp. 893–901.

Five
THE ARMCHAIR WORKOUT
131 **In December 1994, Pam Ruff, a cardiac sonographer . . .** Kathleen Fackelmann, "Diet drug debacle," *Science News*, October 18, 1997, vol. 152, p. 252.
131 **This weight-loss treatment had grown in popularity ever since . . .** Michael Weintraub, "Long-term weight control: National Heart, Lung, and Blood Institute funded Multimodal Intervention Study," *Clinical Pharmacology and Therapeutics*, May 1992, vol. 51, no. 5, pp. 581–646.
133 **Together the doctors from the two medical centers . . .** H. M. Connolly et al., "Valvular heart disease associated with fenfluramine-phentermine," *New England Journal of Medicine*, August 28, 1997, vol. 337, p. 581. L. B. Cannistra, S. M. Davis and A. G. Bauman, "Valvular heart disease associated with dexfenfluramine," *New England Journal of Medicine*, August 28, 1997, vol. 337, p. 636.
133 **At that time, the Food and Drug Administration . . .** http://www.fda.gov/cder/news/phenfennotes, September 17, 1997.
134 **It is an appetite suppressant that slows dissipation . . .** Transcript, Food and Drug Administration Endocrinologic and Metabolic Drugs Advisory Committee meeting 64, Meridia, September 26, 1996. M. E. J. Lean, "Sibutramine—A review of clinical efficacy," *International Journal of Obesity*, 1997, vol. 21, pp. S30–S36.

134 **Close on Meridia's heels in the FDA approval process is Xenical . . .** Transcript, Food and Drug Administration Endocrinologic and Metabolic Drugs Advisory Committee meeting 69, Xenical, March 13, 1998.

135 **By one recent count, 62 new compounds . . .** Interview with Arthur Frank, March 3, 1997.

135 **"I expect we'll see one or two new drugs" . . .** Interview with Leo Lutwak, February 10, 1997.

136 **. . . began to refer to obesity as a disease—a chronic condition . . .** B. T. Burton, W. R. Foster, J. Hirsch, and T. B. Van Itallie, "Health implications of obesity: an NIH Consensus Development Conference," *International Journal of Obesity*, 1985, vol. 9, pp. 155–170.

136 **To that end, NAASO leaders began a quiet campaign . . .** Interview with Judith Stern, March 23, 1997.

137 **Since then, it has jump started the entire field . . .** L. A. Campfield, F. J. Smith, and P. Burn, "The *ob* protein (leptin) pathway—A link between adipose tissue mass and central neural networks," *Hormone and Metabolic Research*, December 1996, vol. 28, pp. 619–632.

138 **In general, people don't become obese because they . . .** Margherita Maffei et al., "Leptin levels in human and rodent: Measurement of plasma leptin and *ob* RNA in obese and weight-reduced subjects," *Nature Medicine*, November 1995, vol. 1, no. 11, pp. 1155–1161.

138 **Experiments in mice support the idea . . .** L. Arthur Campfield, Françoise J. Smith, Yves Guisez, René Devos, and Paul Burn, "Recombinant mouse *ob* protein evidence for a peripheral signal linking adiposity and central neural networks," *Science*, July 28, 1995, vol. 269,

pp. 546–549. Interview with L. Arthur Campfield, August 15, 1995.

139 **In June 1997, Amgen reported that . . .** "Amgen announces leptin causes weight loss in humans and plans for two phase 2 trials," Amgen news release, June 16, 1997.

139 **"That says to me that they were trying to put tons of this material"** . . . Interview with Margaret Van Heek, December 15, 1997.

140 **A study by Andrew Greenberg . . .** Andrew Pollack, "Weight-loss drug shows some success in humans," *The New York Times*, June 15, 1998, p. D7.

140 **"There's this whole series of signals that are integrated"** . . . Interview with L. Arthur Campfield, August 15, 1995.

140 **Leptin and its receptors . . .** C. Streamson, et al., "Phenotypes of mouse *diabetes* and rat *fatty* due to mutations in the *ob* (leptin) receptor," *Science*, February 16, 1996, vol. 271, pp. 994–996. "New chapters in the leptin tale," *Science News*, March 16, 1996, vol. 149, p. 171.

140 **. . . researchers are beginning to see how the many pieces fit together. . . .** Jeffrey M. Friedman, "The alphabet of weight control," *Nature*, January 9, 1997, vol. 385, pp. 119–120. Interview with Friedman, November 11, 1995.

141 **Using these and other examples, Campfield has theorized . . .** L. A. Campfield, F. J. Smith, and P. Burn, "The *ob* protein (leptin) pathway—A link between adipose tissue mass and central neural networks," *Hormone and Metabolic Research*, December 1996, vol. 28, p. 624.

141 **One of their favorite targets has been the beta-3 receptor . . .** Peter Arner, "The (beta)3-adrenergic receptor—A cause and cure of obesity?" *New England Journal of Medicine*, August 10, 1995, vol. 333, no. 6. Interviews with Elliot Danforth, July 16, 1997; Jean Himms-Hagen, July 9, 1997; and anonymous sources within the drug industry.

142 **A handful of drug companies would have had . . .** Alan Connacher et al., "Clinical studies with the beta-adrenoceptor agonist BRL 26830A," *American Journal of Clinical Nutrition*, 1992, vol. 55, pp. 258S–261S.

142 **But the efforts weren't a total waste . . .** Terence T. Yen, "Antiobesity and antidiabetic beta-agonists: Lessons learned and questions to be answered," *Obesity Research*, September 1994, vol. 2, no. 5, pp. 472–480. Terence T. Yen, "Beta-agonists as antiobesity, antidiabetic and nutrient partitioning agents," *Obesity Research*, November 1995, vol. 3, suppl. 4, pp. 531S–536S.

143 **The cloning of that receptor in 1993 put the beta-3 drug program . . .** J. G. Granneman, K. N. Lahners, and A. Chaudhry, "Characterization of the human beta 3-adrenergic receptor gene," *Molecular Pharmacology*, August 1993, vol. 44, no. 2, pp. 264–270.

143 **. . . "really pleased with our development" . . .** Interview with Jamie Dananberg, July 14, 1997.

144 **One day when she was holding her newborn grandson . . .** Interview with Jean Himms-Hagen, July 18, 1997.

144 **The desire of the drug companies to hedge their bets . . .** Trisha Gura, "Uncoupling proteins provide new clue to obesity's causes," *Science*, May 29, 1998, vol. 280, pp. 1369–1370.

145 **The original UCP is only in brown fat . . .** D. Ricquier, L. Casteilla, and F. Bouillaud, "Molecular studies of the uncoupling protein," *FASEB Journal*, June 1991, vol. 5, no. 9, pp. 2237–2242.

145 **UCP2, cloned in March 1997, turns out to be . . .** C. Fleury et al., "Uncoupling protein-2: A novel gene linked to obesity and hyperinsulinemia," *Nature Genetics*, March 1997, vol. 15, no. 3, pp. 269–272.

145 **UCP3, which showed up later the same year . . .** O. Boss et al., "Uncoupling protein-3: A new member of the mitochondrial carrier family with tissue-specific expression," *FEBS Letters*, May 12, 1997, vol. 408, no. 1, pp. 39–42. A. Vidal-Puig et al., "UCP3: An uncoupling protein homologue expressed preferentially and abundantly in skeletal muscle and brown adipose tissue," *Biochemical and Biophysical Research Communications*, June 9, 1997, vol. 235, no. 1, pp. 79–82.

145 **. . . a UCP has been found in potatoes . . .** Maryse Laloi et al., "A plant cold-induced uncoupling protein," *Nature*, September 11, 1997, vol. 389, pp. 135–136.

145 **"The fact that it's in white adipocytes is important" . . .** Interview with Richard Surwit, July 31, 1997.

147 **In a culture where you can scarcely . . .** Interview with Morton Maxwell, August 29, 1996.

148 **What's more, in 1996 a group comprising some of the country's . . .** National Task Force on the Prevention and Treatment of Obesity, "Long-term pharmacotherapy in the management of obesity," *Journal of the American Medical Association*, December 18, 1996, vol. 276, no. 23, pp. 1907–1915.

148 **But Redux and fenfluramine were known to increase the risk of . . .** Norbert F. Voelkel, William R. Clarke, and Timothy Higenbottam, "Obesity, dexfenfluramine,

and pulmonary hypertension: A lesson not learned?" *American Journal of Respiratory and Critical Care Medicine*, 1997, vol. 15, pp. 786–788. Lucien Abenhaim et al., for the International Primary Pulmonary Hypertension Study Group, "Appetite-suppressant drugs and the risk of primary pulmonary hypertension," *New England Journal of Medicine*, August 29, 1996, vol. 335, no. 9, pp. 609–616.

148 **PPH is a condition in which the blood vessels . . .** Lewis J. Rubin, "Primary Pulmonary Hypertension," *Current Concepts*, 1997, vol. 336, no. 2, pp. 111–117.

149 **While taking a prescribed course of these drugs . . .** B. Guy-Grand, M. Apfelbaum, G. Crepaldy, A. Gries, P. Lefebvre, and P. Turner, "International trial of long-term dexfenfluramine in obesity," *Lancet*, 1989, vol. 2, pp. 1142–1144. Michael Weintraub, "Long-term weight control: National Heart, Lung, and Blood Institute funded Multimodal Intervention Study," *Clinical Pharmacology and Therapeutics*, May 1992, vol. 51, no. 5, pp. 581–646.

149 **A handful of obesity researchers, like George Bray . . .** Interview with Bray, July 10, 1996.

150 **What they hope is that drugs will . . .** Interview with Arthur Frank, March 3, 1997.

150 **Meridia induces large, potentially dangerous increases . . .** Transcript, Food and Drug Administration Endocrinologic and Metabolic Drugs Advisory Committee meeting 64, Meridia, September 26, 1996.

150 **After that meeting, Knoll officials convinced the FDA . . .** Interview with Knoll spokesperson Linda Mayer, June 3, 1997.

151 **Curtis Jatkauskas, a Colorado resident who signed on . . .** Interview with Jatkauskas, September 10, 1996.

151 **An even more disturbing problem that stalled . . .** Transcript, Food and Drug Administration Endocrinologic and Metabolic Drugs Advisory Committee meeting 69, Xenical, Friday March 13, 1998. "Anti-obesity pill nears final F.D.A. approval," *The New York Times*, May 15, 1997, p. A20.

152 **Further evidence of those constraints comes from . . .** Interviews with Richard Atkinson, March 10, 1997; Roy Blank, August 29, 1996; Richard A. Lutes, August 29, 1996; John Foreyt, March 5, 1997.

153 **"Food intake is so primary, so central to survival" . . .** Interview with F. Xavier Pi-Sunyer, September 4, 1996.

153 **For these reasons, many researchers believe . . .** R. L. Atkinson, R. C. Blank, J. F. Loper, D. Schumacher, and R. A. Lutes, "Combined drug treatment of obesity," *Obesity Research*, November 1995, vol. 3, suppl. 4, pp. 497s–500s

154 **Combinations of ephedra and caffeine have been studied . . .** A. Astrup, L. Breum, S. Toubro, P. Hein, and F. Quaade, "The effect and safety of an ephedrine/caffeine compound compared to ephedrine, caffeine and placebo in obese subjects on an energy restricted diet: A double blind trial," *International Journal of Obesity*, 1992, vol. 16, pp. 269–277.

155 **Bernard McNamara, director of Weight Control Medical . . .** "The fenfluramine-phentermine phenomenon," *National Association of Boards of Pharmacy Newsletter*, October/November 1995, p. 118.

155 **. . . "is absolutely insane—like saying if you've got" . . .** Interview with Atkinson, March 10, 1997.

157 **With this in mind, thoughtful researchers have begun** . . . Interview with L. Arthur Campfield, August 15, 1985.

157 **. . . Michael Weintraub learned this lesson** . . . Michael Weintraub, "Long-term weight control," p. 644.

158 **"Oh, if you do it seriously enough"** . . . Interview with George Bray, July 10, 1996.

159 **To arguments that diet drugs are being** . . . Interviews with George Bray, July 10, 1996; Bill Dietz, March 10, 1997; Joe Cranston, Director, Department of Drug Policy, American Medical Association, February 10, 1997.

159 **Bray has even gone so far as to write** . . . George A. Bray, "Evaluation of drugs for treating obesity," *Obesity Research*, November 1995, vol. 3, suppl. 4, pp. 425s–434s.

Six
FACING FAT

161 **It is late afternoon in the ballroom** . . . Mardi Gras Fashion Show, NAAFA Annual Convention, July 11, 1996, Hyatt Regency, New Orleans.

163 **In this department, Wann is leading** . . . Marilyn Wann (Ed.), *Fat!So?* 1994–1996, issues 1–6.

164 **Though Wann was launching a fat activist magazine** . . . Wann, "Activism for Everyone," panel discussion at NAAFA Convention, July 11, 1996.

165 **Fat activists don't buy the medical argument that obesity is a chronic** . . . Sally Smith, "Obesity research," *Dimensions*, November 1993, p. 16.

165 **As an example of those attitudes, activists often** . . . Lee Martindale, "Outrage in Chicago: The death and

desecration of Patricia Mullen," *Rump Parliament*, July-August 1996, vol. 5, no. 1, pp. 15–18. "Treatment of obese woman's corpse blasted" by Tara Gruzen, *Chicago Tribune*, May 12 1996, metro p. 1.

167 **. . . such constant negative input can have a profound effect . . .** Lisa Schoenfelder and Barb Wieser (Eds.), *Shadows on a Tightrope: Writings by Women on Fat Oppression* (Aunt Lute Book Company, 1983).

167 **"Because when you go out in public at a heavy weight" . . .** Interview with Ellen Gordon, July 9, 1996.

168 **. . . sees that group's local and national meetings as . . .** Francis White, opening remarks at NAAFA Convention, July 9, 1996.

168 **In some cases, the effort to normalize size has led . . .** "A starting point for change and renewal," *NAAFA Newsletter*, February/March 1996, vol. 26, no. 1, p. 7.

169 **One of the most important health issues for obese people . . .** "Dispelling Common Myths About Fat People," pamphlet put out by NAAFA.

169 **Surveys of the medical community have repeatedly . . .** G. L. Maddox and P. C. Liederman, "Overweight and social desirability with medical implications," *Journal of Medical Education*, March 1969, vol. 44, no. 3, pp. 214–220. L. M. Breytspraak et al., "Sensitizing medical students to impression formation processes in the patient interview," *Journal of Medical Education*, 1977, vol. 52, pp. 47–54.

169 **. . . A more recent study . . .** J. H. Price, S. M. Desmond, R. A. Krol, F. F. Snyder, and J. K. O'Connell, "Family practice physicians' beliefs, attitudes and practices regarding obesity," *American Journal of Preventive Medicine*, 1987, vol. 3, pp. 339–345. Arthur Frank, "Futility and avoidance:

Medical professionals in the treatment of obesity," *Journal of the American Medical Association*, April 28, 1993, vol. 269, no. 16, pp. 2132–2133.

170 **Activists are well-versed in the multiple conflicts . . .** Sally Smith, "The great diet deception," *USA Today*, January 1995, pp. 76–78.

170 **This isn't to say that size activists would put an end . . .** "Leptin touted as 'miracle Cure,'" *NAAFA Newsletter*, July/August 1995, vol. 25, no. 6, p. 1.

171 **To redress these problems, NAAFA has issued . . .** "Declaration of the Rights of Fat People in Health Care," pamphlet put out by NAAFA.

172 **National diet programs like Nutri/System and Jenny Craig . . .** Leslie Vreeland, "Lean times in fat city," *Working Woman*, July 1995, pp. 47–74.

172 **Medical professionals have also begun to suggest . . .** Jerome Kassirer and Marcia Angell, "Losing weight— An ill-fated New Year's resolution," *New England Journal of Medicine*, January 1, 1998, vol. 338, no. 1, pp. 52–54.

173 **"We're determined that we're not going to pay again" . . .** Interview with Lynn McAfee, March 7, 1997.

174 **. . . rumors that were started by a flippant remark . . .** "Cass Elliot, pop singer, dies; star of the Mamas and Papas," *The New York Times*, July 30, 1974, p. 36.

174 **In fact, an autopsy of the singer by two British doctors . . .** "Cass Elliot's death linked to heart attack," *The New York Times*, August 6, 1974, p. 39.

Seven
IN DEFERENCE TO DIFFERENCE

177 **"I said, 'Hold on a minute. You're telling me'" . . .** Interview with Nikhil Dhurandhar, January 16, 1998.

177 **When the two men took 20 chickens and injected . . .** N. V. Dhurandhar, P. R. Kulkarni, S. M. Ajinkya, and A. A. Sherikar, "Effect of adenovirus infection on adiposity in chickens," *Veterinary Microbiology*, 1992, vol. 31, pp. 101–107.

178 **Dhurandhar couldn't help but wonder whether people . . .** Nikhil V. Dhurandhar et al., "Association of adenovirus infection with human obesity," *Obesity Research*, September 1997, vol. 5, no. 5, pp. 464–469.

178 **He knew that avian adenoviruses weren't supposed . . .** G. Mlinaric-Galinovic, I. Ugrcic, D. Detic, and J. Bozikov, "Epidemiological picture of viral infections in Croatia," *Acta Medica Iugoslavica*, 1991, vol. 45, pp. 203–211.

178 **. . . until the Hong Kong bird flu . . .** Kanta Subbarao et al., "Characterization of an avian influenza A (H5N1) virus isolated from a child with a fatal respiratory illness," *Science*, January 16, 1998, vol. 279, pp. 393–396.

179 **. . . Atkinson has been interested in obesity viruses ever since he read a 1982 paper . . .** Michael J. Lyons, Irving M. Faust, Richard B. Hemmes, Daniel R. Buskirk, Jules Hirsch, and John B. Zabriskie, "A virally induced obesity syndrome in mice," *Science*, April 2, 1982, vol. 216, pp. 82–85. Interview with Atkinson, February 11, 1998.

181 **The human obesity virus, while plausible . . .** Dhurandhar's best theory is that this is a GI tract virus, spread by coming into contact with feces, for example. It was isolated from the feces of a diabetic girl. If this is the case, then according to Dhurandhar, good hand washing may currently be the best way to avoid getting such a virus. He and Atkinson are at work on a vaccine.

182   **Viruses are implicated in several types of cancer . . .**
Harald zur Hausen, "Viruses in human cancers,
Science, November 22, 1991, vol. 254, pp. 1167–1172.

182   **. . . atherosclerosis . . .** Sandra Blakeslee, "Common
virus seen as having early role in arteries' clogging," *The
New York Times,* January 29, 1991, p. C3.

182   **. . . and mood disorders . . .** L. Bode, W. Zimmermann,
R. Ferszt, F. Steinbach, and H. Ludwig, "Borna disease
virus genome transcribed and expressed in psychiatric
patients," *Nature Medicine,* March 1995, vol. 1, no. 3,
pp. 232–236.

182   **The number of people in the United States who fit
the . . .** Robert Kuczmarski et al., "Increasing prevalence of overweight among U.S. adults: National Health
and Nutrition Examination Surveys, 1960 to 1991,"
Journal of the American Medical Association, July 20
1994, vol. 272, no. 3, pp. 205–211.

184   **Researchers once hoped . . .** Atkinson, February 11,
1998.

185   **In the most recent update, Bouchard identified 75
genes . . .** Yvon C. Chagnon, Louis Perusse, and Claude
Bouchard, "The human obesity gene map: 1997
update," *Obesity Research,* January 1998, vol. 6, no. 1,
pp. 76–92.

186   **One of the researchers who has consistently . . .** Eric
Ravussin and P. Antonio Tataranni, "Dietary fat and
human obesity," *Journal of the American Dietetic
Association,* July 1997, vol. 97, no. 7, suppl. 7,
pp. S42–S46.

186   **In a decade of work, Ravussin has uncovered . . .**
Eric Ravussin, "Predictors of weight gain from physiology to genetics," *Obesity Research,* October 3, 1995, vol. 3,
suppl. 3, p. 317s.

187 **In one study of more than 500 Pima volunteers . . .**
Pietro A. Tataranni and Eric Ravussin, "Variability in metabolic rate: Biological sites of regulation," *International Journal of Obesity*, 1995, vol. 19, suppl. 4, pp. S102–S106.

187 **The researchers gathered this information using . . .**
Clifton Bogardus et al., "Familial dependence of the resting metabolic rate," *New England Journal of Medicine*, July 10, 1986, vol. 315, no. 2, p. 97. Henry Montoye et al. (Eds.), *Measuring Physical Activity and Energy Expenditure* (Human Kinetics, 1996) pp. 4–8.

188 **"Most of the obese patients you see" . . .** Interview with Eric Ravussin, February 11, 1998.

189 **A low metabolic rate can, of course, contribute . . .**
Eric Ravussin et al., "Reduced rate of energy expenditure as a risk factor for body-weight gain," *New England Journal of Medicine*, February 25, 1988, vol. 318, no. 8, pp. 467–472.

190 **That's the explanation favored by Colorado obesity researcher . . .** Interview with James Hill, September 10, 1996.

190 **Human variety influences the effectiveness of obesity treatment . . .** Gary D. Foster et al., "Resting energy expenditure, body composition, and excess weight in the obese," *Metabolism*, May 1988, vol. 37, no. 5, pp. 467–472.

191 **In a conference on exercise and obesity . . .** Exercise and Obesity: Morphological, Metabolic and Clinical Implications: A Satellite Symposium of the 7th International Congress on Obesity, August 17–19, 1994, Quebec city, Canada.

191 **. . . chose to devote his talk to this topic . . .** Claude Bouchard, "Individual differences in the response to

regular exercise," *International Journal of Obesity*, 1995, vol. 19, suppl. 4, pp. S5–S7.

194 **"Human beings vary on every single trait"** . . . Interview with Steven Blair, June 23, 1997.

194 **. . . "you're right back to that statement of the American College"** . . . Russell R. Pate et al., "Physical activity and public health: A recommendation from the Centers for Disease Control and Prevention and the American College of Sports Medicine," *Journal of the American Medical Association*, February 1, 1995, vol. 273, no. 5, pp. 402–407.

196 **Stories of people who lost 30 or 40 pounds** . . . Michael Lemonick, "The new miracle drug?" *Time*, September 21, 1996, pp. 61–67. Interview with John Foreyt, March 5, 1997.

196 **The same variety of effects can be found** . . . M. E. J. Lean, "Clinical efficacy of sibutramine," *International Journal of Obesity*, 1997, vol. 21, suppl. 1, pp. S30–S36. B. Guy-Grand, M. Stock, M. Lean, and A. Astrup, "Discussion Panel 2: The role of sibutramine in the treatment of obesity," *International Journal of Obesity*, 1997, vol. 21, suppl. 1, pp. S37–S39.

196 **"That's my main issue when you look at the future"** . . . Interview with Lynn McAfee, March 7, 1997.

197 **Obesity researchers put it in slightly more technical** . . . Interview with David West, February 5, 1997.

197 **Similar screening tests are already being developed** . . . "Pharmacogenomics: Revolution or Reaction," a roundtable discussion at the BIO'98 International Biotechnology Meeting and Exhibition, June 16, 1998. Lawrence M. Fisher, "Smoother road from lab to sales," *The New York Times*, February 25, 1998, p. D1.

Eight
WADDLING TOWARDS BETHLEHEM

199 **Every year on the last Saturday in August . . .**
Interview with Crooked River Mitch, August 13, 1996.

203 **The woman's question brought to my mind . . .** L. L.
Birch, "Children's food intake: A developmental perspective," *Obesity Research*, October 3, 1995, vol. 3,
suppl. 3, p. 307s.

203 **"Left to their own devices" . . .** Susan L. Johnson and
Leann L. Birch, "Parents' and children's adiposity and eating style," *Pediatrics*, November 1994, vol. 94, no. 5, pp.
653–661. Interview with Leann Birch, February 16, 1995.

205 **Six months before that flight, I was sitting in a lec-
ture hall . . .** "Overweight America: Strategies for
Change," symposium at the Harvard School of Public
Health, May 1, 1995. Moderated by Steve Gortmaker.
Speakers: Walter Willett, Bill Dietz, Aviva Must.

205 **Such social issues have been at the heart of
Gortmaker's research . . .** S. L. Gortmaker, W. H.
Dietz, Jr., and L. W. Cheung, "Inactivity, diet, and the
fattening of America," *Journal of the American Dietetic
Association*, September 1990, vol. 90, no. 9,
pp. 1247–1252.

206 **Children seem to be particularly vulnerable to these
effects . . .** S. L. Gortmaker, A. Must, A. M. Sobel, K.
Peterson, G. A. Colditz, and W. H. Dietz, "Television
viewing as a cause of increasing obesity among children
in the United States, 1986–1990," *Archives of Pediatrics
and Adolescent Medicine*, April 1996, vol. 150, no. 4,
pp. 356–362.

207 **A good example of what Dietz means comes from . . .**
L. H. Epstein, A. M. Valoski, L. S. Vara, J. McCurley,

L. Wisniewski, M. A. Kalarchian, K. R. Klein, and L. R. Shrager, "Effects of decreasing sedentary behavior and increasing activity on weight change in obese children," *Health Psychology*, 1995, vol. 14, no. 2, pp. 109–115.

207 **Because Epstein's previous studies have shown . . .** Leonard H. Epstein, Alice Valoski, Rena R. Wing, and James McCurley, "Ten-year follow-up of behavioral, family-based treatment for obese children," *Journal of the American Medical Association*, November 21, 1990, vol. 264, no. 19, pp. 2519–2523.

210 **Such was the thrust of a January 1, 1998, editorial . . .** Jerome Kassirer and Marcia Angell, "Losing weight— An ill-fated New Year's resolution," *New England Journal of Medicine*, January 1, 1998, vol. 338, no. 1, pp. 52–54.

210 **In the months after its publication . . .** Theodore van Itallie, "Excess Morbidity and Mortality Attributable to Overweight," lecture at Harvard Medical School, May 13, 1998.

211 **"No matter where you are in the population" . . .** Comments of Bill Dietz at symposium, "Overweight America: Strategies for Change."

211 **Some of the most interesting research . . .** B. C. Hansen and N. L. Bodkin, "Primary prevention of diabetes mellitus by prevention of obesity in monkeys," *Diabetes*, December 1993, vol. 42, no. 12, pp. 1809–1814. B. C. Hansen, H. K. Ortmeyer, and B. L. Bodkin, "Prevention of obesity in middle-aged monkeys: Food intake during body weight clamp," *Obesity Research*, September 1995, vol. 3, suppl. 2, pp. 199s–204s.

211 **"I like to refer to it as the bathroom scale model" . . .** Interview with Barbara Hansen, August 28, 1996.

Index